The Squat Bible

The Ultimate Guide to Mastering the Squat and Finding Your True Strength

Dr. Aaron Horschig
Founder of Squat University

with

Dr. Kevin Sonthana
and
Travis Neff

Copyright © 2016 Dr. Aaron Horschig
All rights reserved.

This book is for educational purposes only. The publisher and the authors are not responsible for any adverse harmful effects arising as a result of the information provided. The exercises described in this book should be used with caution and practiced safely. Always consult with a medical professional before attempting to perform these movements and starting a workout program.

ISBN 13: 9781095696958 (paperback)
Library of Congress Control Number: 2016919281
LCCN Imprint Name: **Squat University LLC**

Contents

Preface vii

Chapter 1   A Movement First, an Exercise Second 1
            1.1 The Looking Glass of Movement 1
            1.2 Learning How to Squat
                 (Bodyweight Squat) 7
                 1.2.1 The Absolutes of Squatting 8
                 1.2.2 The Bodyweight Squat 17

Chapter 2   Barbell Squat Technique 21
            2.1 Maintaining Postural Integrity 21
                 2.1.1 Core Stability 22
                 2.1.2 Proper Breathing 24
            2.2 The High-Bar Back Squat 29
            2.3 The Low-Bar Back Squat 37
            2.4 The Front Squat 43
            2.5 The Overhead Squat 50

Chapter 3   The Joint-by-Joint Concept 59

Chapter 4   The Stable Foot 69

Chapter 5	The Mobile Ankle	73
	5.1 Screening for Ankle Stiffness	73
	5.2 Joint Restriction or Soft-Tissue Stiffness?	76
	5.3 Mobility Corner	80
Chapter 6	The Stable Knee	87
	6.1 Screening for Knee Instability	89
	6.2 Corrective Exercise Corner	90
Chapter 7	The Mobile Hip	98
	7.1 Screening for Hip Stiffness	99
	7.2 Joint Restriction or Soft-Tissue Stiffness?	101
	7.3 Mobility Corner	105
Chapter 8	The Stable Core	114
	8.1 Level 1 (Cognitive Stability)	115
	8.2 Level 2 (Movement Stability)	117
	8.3 Level 3 (Functional Stability)	120
Chapter 9	Overhead Mobility	124
	9.1 Screening Overhead Mobility	124
	9.2 Mobility Corner	129
Chapter 10	The Stable Shoulder Blade	139
	10.1 Screening for Scapular Instability	140
	10.2 Corrective Exercise Corner	141

Chapter 11	Debunking Squat Myths.. 148
	11.1 Are Deep Squats Bad for Your Knees?.... 148
	11.2 Should My Knees Go Past My Toes?........ 157
	11.3 Toes Forward or Angled Out?.................. 164

Chapter 12	The Real Science of the Squat 172
	12.1 Squat Biomechanics................................... 173
	12.2 Squat Analysis 1.0....................................... 177
	12.3 Squat Analysis 2.0....................................... 187

Acknowledgments 197

Preface

I often find myself experiencing flashes of déjà vu. I'll be talking with athletes who are complaining of pain. They'll explain how their knees or backs hurt when they move this way or that. By the time they've come to me, they've usually exhausted almost every avenue of self-treatment one can find via Google search. Ice baths, pain meds, electrical stimulation; I've heard it all. Athletes will try anything to keep their athletic performance from faltering.

We'll eventually arrive at the crossroads in our conversation where I ask, "Okay, let me see what your squat looks like." Typically, at this point the once free-flowing conversation sputters to a direct halt. I'm met with a perplexed look as if the athletes are expecting a more scientific medical examination. Eventually the athletes will rise from their chairs, face me, set their feet…and it begins.

When I first started writing this book, I was often met with the question, "Why write a book on squatting?" Instantly dozens of answers ran through my head. The one answer that came to me is that "the squat is the building block to finding your true strength."

The ancient Greek philosopher Socrates once wrote, "No man has the right to be an amateur in the matter of physical training. It is a shame for a man to go through life without finding the true strength he is capable of."

When most of us first think about *strength*, we instantly picture a colossal athlete lifting tremendous weight. I usually envision the bodybuilding monster Ronnie Coleman. He was famous for his weight-training antics that spurred millions of YouTube views. My friends and I would constantly replay videos of Ronnie screaming, "*Yeah, Buddy!*" (loudly enough for the whole weight room to hear). He would literally throw hundred-pound dumbbells as if they were plastic toys. There is no denying Ronnie is strong. In many ways, he is the American definition of strength.

Today we live in a performance-driven society. There's no question about it. Everything from the workplace to the athletic field is judged and graded on how *much* we can accomplish. How *much* we can perform.

On ESPN, we are constantly barraged with physical highlights. Who ran the fastest forty-yard dash? Who lifted the latest world-record weight? Who hit the most homeruns?

The way athletes live, train, and compete today echoes our performance-driven society. We base *everything* on the mantra of becoming bigger, faster, and stronger.

Unfortunately, there is an ugly flip side to this approach. Every single year, thousands of athletes around the world suffer traumatic season-ending injuries. Experts estimate over one hundred thousand young athletes will tear their ACL in the United States alone this year. The scary thing is that the rate of these injuries is only growing.

In our pursuit of physical-performance accolades, we have lost sight of our athletes' movement capabilities. We have rearranged our athletic priorities to such an extent that only our performance matters to many. In doing so, we have successfully capsized many athletes' potential and brought upon this injury epidemic.

You see, the problem isn't that athletes today are too big, or too strong, or too fast. The issue is that athletes have become so in a way that is not supported by enough quality movement. Therein lays the problem. Too many athletes today are moving poorly.

The foundation from which performance potential is built upon is the same one that also supports and keeps an athlete injury-free. In reality, strength and conditioning professionals and sports-medicine practitioners have a common language. This is the language of movement. Instead of turning to complicated research and pricey technology, we need to take a step back and address the cornerstone of our movement foundation.

Without mastery of the simplest movement patterns, there is no way to reach the peak physical potential Socrates was writing about. Until we change our perspective and become masters of our physical bodies by moving *better* before we try to move *more*, we will continue to fall short of our potential. And we will continue to see a rise in injuries. These changes all start with the squat.

In the following pages, you will find a simple way to assess your squatting movement and understand how to fix these problems before injury occurs. After mastering the bodyweight squat, you will then learn how to perfect the exercise of the barbell squat.

When Steve Jobs introduced the world to the Apple I, he did so with the desire to put the power of the personal computer in each individual's hands. By empowering the individual in this technological way, he was able to change the world.

The same empowerment can be found through the teachings in this book. Let me use a real-life example to help solidify this point. Recently I was having a discussion with a young Olympic weightlifter. She was telling me how she had been dealing with knee pain for the past few weeks every time she squatted, cleaned, or snatched the barbell. I asked her what she had been doing to help fix the pain. She replied, "I've iced my knees, stretched my quads, and rested."

She went on that the pain had gotten so bad that she had even had to modify her normal training schedule. Her performance was beginning to suffer, and her coach was not happy to say the least. To make things worse, she had a national-level competition in a few weeks. She was at her wits' end.

When she asked if I thought I could help her knees, I smiled and nodded my head. Without hesitation, we started our examination to find out the cause of her pain. Yet again, I found myself in the same situation I seemingly end up in time and time again. Was it déjà vu?

As the conversation sputtered to a halt, I uttered the question, "Okay, let me see what your squat looks like." Welcome to Squat University. Let's begin.

Chapter 1
A Movement First, an Exercise Second

1.1 The Looking Glass of Movement

If I had one goal for this book, it would be to inspire you to look at the body in a different manner. I want you to take a step back from conventional wisdom and the ways in which we have viewed and analyzed the body in the past. It's time to take off the blinders and really understand our bodies through a new medium: the looking glass of human movement.

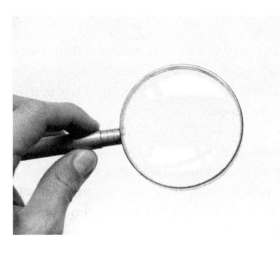

Today we live in a performance-driven culture. Every year *Fortune* magazine boasts the famous Fortune 500 list, ranking the top five hundred corporations in the United States based solely on their total revenue. Our current paradigm is centered on what we can achieve and accomplish if we just do X, Y, and Z. It's no wonder that the American win-at-all-cost culture has penetrated every aspect of our lives—including sports.

The mantra "Bigger, Faster, Stronger" is echoed in every aspect of sport performance today. The idea of lifting more weight, running the faster time, and setting the next record has consumed us for decades—a testament to who we are as a society. Has it been effective? You bet. Just look at the 2012 Olympic Games and search for how many world records were set. The answer is thirty-two new world records. However, even after all of the performance advances we have made over the past years, the faster times, the more weight lifted, and the increased yardage ran, there was still something missing. Despite the accolades and honors, athletes kept getting injured at an alarming rate.

For example, injury to the anterior cruciate ligament (ACL) has been labeled as one of the most serious season-ending injuries in all of sports today. Let me throw up a few numbers to explain this phenomenon.

- An estimated one hundred thousand ACL tears will happen this year in the United States.[1]
- Nearly two-thirds of these injuries are noncontact—meaning the injury did not involve any contact with another player.[2,3]

- Girls who play soccer and basketball are currently tearing their ACL three times more than boys are.[4]
- Research has shown that roughly 5 percent of all girls who play year-round basketball and soccer will sustain a tear to their ACL at some point in their career.[4]

You see, the issue is not that our athletes are too big, too fast, or too strong—those are all part of normal human evolution in a performance-driven society—but it is that they have become so in a way that is not supported by their fundamental movement foundation. Ask yourself if any of these situations sound familiar to you.

- You notice a large powerlifter at your gym who can squat seven hundred pounds in the back squat but struggles to perform a basic front squat because of his poor mobility restrictions.
- You know a football player with knee pain—he can back squat five hundred pounds but cannot perform a basic pistol squat without his knee wobbling around uncontrollably.
- You observe a weightlifter who can clean and jerk four hundred pounds but allows his knees to roll in on the ascent portion of the clean movement.
- A strength coach tells you that learning how to perform a pistol squat is a waste of your time because you will never need to get into that position playing football.

Anyone? Unfortunately, these situations are all-too-common occurrences in our culture of performance.

What if I told you we could eliminate roughly seventy thousand torn ACL injuries every year by teaching our athletes how to squat properly? As a doctor of physical therapy, I have the opportunity on a daily basis to observe the quality of movement with athletes of all ages and skill sets. Working at Boost Physical Therapy & Sport Performance in Kansas City, I have been able to accumulate over ten thousand hours in contact time understanding and rehabilitating athletes with this devastating injury. From the high-school female soccer player to the NFL cornerback, there is one constant that connects them all.

For a young female soccer player, a torn ACL can be extremely debilitating, both physically and mentally. A season-ending injury like this eliminates roughly 25 percent of that athlete's high-school career. Competitive soccer today is one of the most popular and time-demanding sports for today's youth. It is common for an athlete of this caliber to donate a minimum of six hours every single week to participating in numerous practices and games. A typical schedule for a competitive soccer player would include three two-hour practices a week, two one-hour sessions of skill work on top of practice, all followed by two or three one-hour-long games every single weekend. Playing at this level demands a high level of skill, and most youth at this level spend hours every week improving their ability to play the sport they love.

The NFL is full of the nation's best athletes—hands down. Only a select few are lucky and talented enough to don an NFL jersey and stand on the sidelines on Sunday afternoon. Less than 1 percent of high-school football players will eventually make it to the NFL. They are big, they are strong, and they are extremely fast. The NFL is quintessentially the pillar of elite athleticism in American society. At this level, performance on the field can mean the difference between being cut and sent home or getting a million-dollar deal and company endorsements that will set a player up for a lifetime of financial stability. An ACL tear therefore can be extremely damaging—physically, mentally, and financially.

While both of these athletes sustained this same injury at different stages in their sporting careers, they also had one common connection that is usually less recognized: They could not squat well. They could not perform a deep bodyweight squat with adequate ankle and hip mobility, proper joint alignment, or muscular coordination. A large majority of each of their rehabilitation was spent learning how to perform a bodyweight squat and a single-leg pistol squat. Most people would think these athletes, both advanced in skill within their respective sports, would be able to perform these simple movements with ease.

The case I'm trying to make with these two athletes is the same phenomenon I see with almost every single athlete I have seen who has sustained the same injury. These athletes didn't sustain their injury because they are weak. These two athletes, just like the thousands that sustain the same ACL tear every single year, spend hours upon hours during the week at the gym or on the training field working on improving their physical capacity to run faster, jump higher, and lift more weight. We as a society value quantity and objective numbers over quality and process. Too often, we place too much emphasis how much weight is on the bar when the athlete can't even perform a basic bodyweight squat or pistol squat to full depth without falling over.

Our performance-driven culture has placed such an emphasis on performance that we have conceptually rearranged our athletic priorities. More often than not athletes are willing to sacrifice movement in order to perform. After all is said and done, we cannot escape the need for movement competency. This concept of movement competency can be described as the ability for an individual to move without pain or discomfort and with proper joint alignment, muscular coordination, and posture.[4]

Now, I'm not saying that the grind of training for performance is not important. What I am saying is that we need to ensure our physical capacity (our strength, our power, our endurance) and our skills do not exceed our ability to move. This starts by solidifying the foundation for our athletic bodies, starting with movement competency. Being able to show competency in our fundamental and functional movement patterns, such as our ability to perform a deep squat with correct joint alignment and muscular coordination, creates a foundation for which strength and skill are predicated upon. Food for thought: Barbell training is one of the most important ways in which we can challenge our body to maintain competency and integrity of our functional movement patterns. Move first and perform second.

If we are unable to move efficiently with good technique in the squat (especially without a barbell), we essentially set ourselves up for failure. Performance-wise, we limit our potential to produce efficient force and power. We also increase our susceptibility to injury because our physical capacity is resting on a faulty platform of fundamental movement.

Regardless of how big, fast, or strong we are, we require a fundamental base of movement. With this fundamental base, we can ensure that what we are gaining in strength and skill when we train can be maintained safely and efficiently. The cornerstone of this foundation is rooted in one simple movement: the squat.

It's like building a house without a proper foundation. You could build a beautiful house that's filled with expensive furnishings in each and every room. This house may even seem secure and sound from an outsider's perspective. However, an inexperienced person with little knowledge of architecture can tell you the house built on a faulty base is set up for eventual failure. Proper functioning of our physical "house" requires that we move first with movement competency before we perform.

Instead of adapting to our limitations or just ignoring them all together, it's time to fix our movement issues. It's time to shift our training efforts that have been focused on remodeling our physical house without ever fixing the large crack in our home's foundation. This starts with seeing the athlete in a different manner—through the looking glass of movement.

1.2 Learning How to Squat (Bodyweight Squat)

When we talk about the squat, many people often want to jump right into discussing the barbell squat. We forget the basics of the bodyweight squat. If we don't address the movement of the squat before the exercise version of the squat, we set ourselves up for failure.

If we can fix the issues that present themselves during the

bodyweight squat, we give ourselves a greater capability to carry the load of the barbell. We should all have the ability to perform a full-depth "ass-to-grass" squat without any weight. Period.

We all want to live, play, and compete in a pain-free manner for as long as we live. This starts with learning how to squat correctly with the bodyweight movement.

1.2.1 The Absolutes of Squatting

In this chapter, we will discuss the five absolutes of squatting. It doesn't matter how tall you are, your level of weight-room experience, or your goals with sport training. These absolutes must be followed in order to squat correctly and remain pain free.

Toe Angle

Most people have a pretty good idea of what the perfect squat looks like in the bottom position. What if I told you that the setup and movement of the squat are actually more important than the bottom position itself?

A common misconception is that people should place their feet at the exact same width during the squat. The width of our stance is *not* one of the absolutes of squatting. Most people are going to have slight differences in how wide they place their feet. Individual mobility limitations and anatomical differences will impact the width of your stance. The goal is to place your feet in a position that will allow for a full-depth squat and still feel comfortable. That being said, placing your feet at around a shoulder width is a good starting position for most.

The stance you assume should be able to carry over to a number of other movements you may perform throughout your day or on the field of play as an athlete. This is the reason why the squat has been called a functional movement. Think about the defensive "ready position" of the basketball player or that of a third baseman just before the pitcher winds up. The starting stance of the squatting movement is a universal position that carries over into many other movement patterns. For this reason, we want to use a fairly straightforward foot position to start this bodyweight squat.

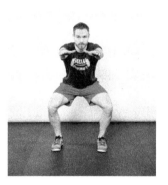

A near straightforward foot position with a very slight five- to seven-degrees out-toe angle during the bodyweight squat is ideal. If you have difficulty performing the movement to full range with this foot position, it may indicate you have certain issues in mobility that warrant attention. This is our first absolute of the bodyweight squat.

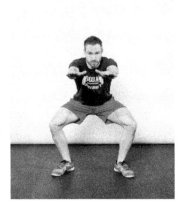

Some coaches will cue their athletes to squat with a much greater angle of out-toeing during the bodyweight squat. Teaching athletes to set up in this manner will likely carry over to other movement patterns that are derived from the squat.

You probably will never see a good linebacker stand in his "ready" position with his toes turned out like a duck. This position is not only inefficient but it also increases risk of injury. That linebacker will not be able to move quickly from this position or unleash an extreme amount of power into his next tackle with his feet turned out.

For the bodyweight squat, a straightforward position is ideal. For the barbell squat, it's acceptable and desirable to toe out a bit more. This will allow a lifter to descend to a greater depth and increase stability. The specifics of the barbell squat movement will be a topic of another chapter.

The Tripod Foot

Once we have our toe-out angle set, let's discuss what we're doing with our feet. When we create a good arch in our feet, we inevitably form what we call a "tripod" foot.

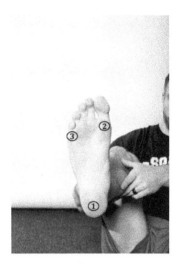

The three points of the tripod consist of the heel, the base of the first toe, and the base of the fifth toe. Our foot is basically like a three-wheeled motorcycle. Our goal when squatting should be to maintain the arch of our feet and have our weight distributed evenly. If all of the wheels are in contact with the ground, we get more power. If one wheel is off the ground or if the body bottoms out, power is lost and the motorcycle breaks down. When our foot is out of position (arch collapse), stability and power are lost.

Distributing the body's weight over the three points of contact of the foot allows for the most efficient base of support possible. Mastering the tripod foot is the second absolute of squatting.

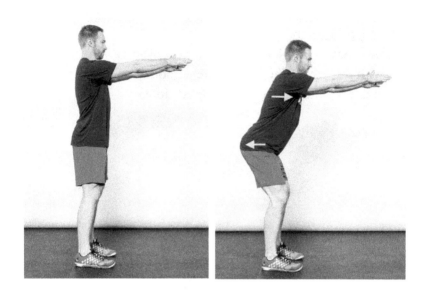

Hip Hinge

Once we have established a comfortable foot position (as close to straightforward as possible and in a tripod position), we are ready for our next step and cue: drive the hips back.

Every squat must start with a hip hinge. By driving our hips backward and bringing the chest forward in a hinging movement, the posterior chain (glutes and hamstrings) is properly engaged.

The hips are the powerhouse of our body. During the squat, these specific muscles drive us up and out of the hole, allowing us to lift tremendous weights. It is therefore imperative to make sure these muscles are used efficiently. This establishes our third absolute of squatting.

Creating External Rotation Torque

Our last cue before starting our descent for the bodyweight squat is to create external rotational torque at the hips. Creating this tension creates a springlike tightness in our hips that will ensure our knees track with ideal alignment during the entire squat.

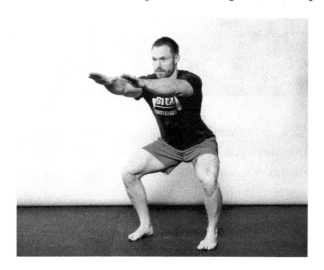

To create this torque at the hips, I use the cues to "squeeze your glutes" and "drive the knees out." In performing these actions, we essentially wind up the springlike mechanism of our hips. If you try this, you will instantly feel the outside muscles of your hips engage. Immediately, the knees will be drawn into a good position in line with the toes, and an arch will be created in the foot.

If we look at the arch of our foot, we notice that it moves in relation to the rest of our lower body. If the knees bow outward, the entire foot moves into a full arched position. When the knees fall inward, the foot subsequently collapses and the arch flattens out. For this reason, the correct position for our lower body can be achieved by the proper action of our hips.

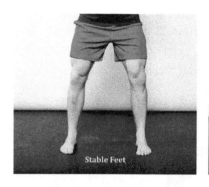
Stable Feet

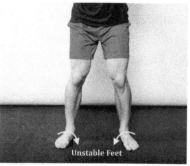
Unstable Feet

We have to remember not to compromise the tripod foot during this step. For this reason, make sure not to push the knees out too far. Some athletes will misuse the cue to drive their knees too far out to the side. Doing this will cause the foot to lose stability and roll on the outside. The goal is to align the knees with the toes. Creating this rotational torque at the hips is the fourth absolute of squatting.

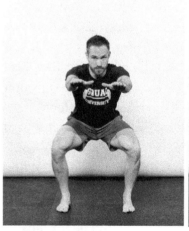
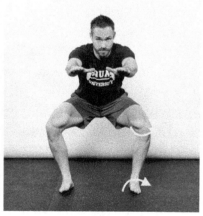

Postural Integrity
Correct technique in the squat relies on every part of our body working in perfect coordination. This includes maintaining our trunk and neck in a neutral and straight position. The concept of postural integrity is our fifth and final absolute.

In order to remain balanced during the squat, we require our center of gravity to be over the middle of our feet. This requires a more forward chest position. However, just because the trunk is required to lean forward does not mean our chest should collapse as if we have a turtle shell on our back.

A cue that can help maintain the ideal straight-trunk position is to hold the arms straight out in front of the body. By holding our arms out in front of our body, our trunk naturally assumes a straighter position.

Maintaining a neutral neck position will depend on the angle of the torso. During the bodyweight squat, our trunk is usually inclined forward over our knees. This requires the athlete to look forward or slightly down (at a point ten to fifteen feet forward on the ground). If the trunk is required to be in a more vertical position (front squat or overhead squat), eye gaze can now be focused more forward or even slightly up (at a point five feet above the horizontal).

Review Time
Let's now review our five absolutes for the bodyweight squat.

1. Point your feet relatively straightforward. Five- to seven-degree toe-out angle is normal.

2. Maintain three points of contact with your feet in relation to the floor, establishing the tripod foot.
3. Hip hinge to engage the posterior chain (glutes and hamstrings) by pushing your hips backward slightly and bringing your chest forward. Your bodyweight should be balanced over the middle of your feet.
4. Create external rotational torque at the hips by squeezing your glutes and shoving the knees out to the side while maintaining the tripod foot.
5. Solidify your postural integrity by holding your arms out in front (parallel to the floor) while looking straight ahead.

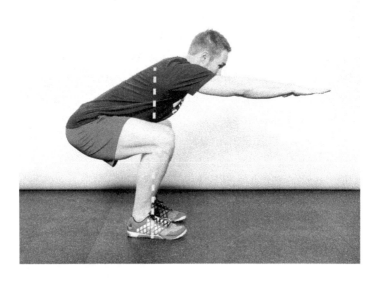

1.2.2 The Bodyweight Squat

The Descent

Once you have accomplished the five absolutes, you can start the descent toward the bottom of the squat. Don't think about stopping high or dropping too low. Just descend into the bottommost position your mobility will allow. Make sure to stay balanced the entire movement. It is important to use this time to feel for where your weight is being held over your feet. This ability to sense body position is called proprioception.

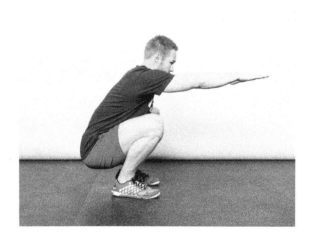

During the descent try to keep the shins in a vertical position for as long as possible. When we fail to keep our shins as vertical as possible for as long as possible, the knees begin to move forward over the toes too soon. This premature forward movement increases forces on the knee joint and leaves the athlete off balance.

Bottom Position

When you have reached full depth in the squat, you should feel solid and completely balanced. Your weight should be evenly distributed between the front and back of your feet. If we drew a vertical line from your body's center of gravity in this position, it should run right through the middle of your foot.

The Ascent

Standing up from the bottom of the squat is all about hip drive. This is accomplished by pushing the hips up and backward. While driving the hips, also visualize pulling your shins back to a vertical position. Doing this allows for efficient use of the posterior chain. This takes pressure off the knees and places the muscles of the hip in a position to create tremendous force. Make sure the chest rises at the same rate as the hips. If the hips rise too quickly, the chest will reflexively fall forward and your body will be off balance.

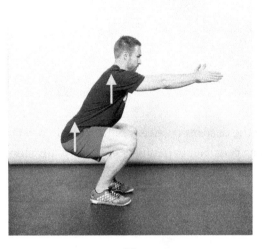

During the ascent of the squat, the knees need to stay in a stable position. This means keeping the knees in line with the feet throughout the entire movement. Improving this control allows us to avoid injury while increasing the efficiency of our movement. By increasing the efficiency of our movements, we increase the potential to produce more power and increase strength. Who wouldn't want more power, more strength, and meanwhile avoid injuries?

Take Away
The bodyweight squat is often a movement passed over by athletes and coaches. Too often, we assume we have the capacity to perform a perfect squat. Don't take for granted that anyone can perform this movement just because he or she is athletic. The squat is a movement first and an exercise second.

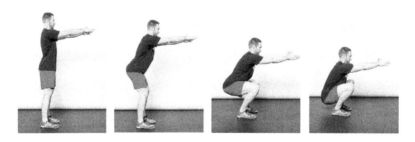

Notes

1. C. C. Prodromos, Y. Han, J. Rogowski, et al., "A Meta-analysis of the Incidence of Anterior Cruciate Ligament Tears as a Function of Gender, Sport, and a Knee Injury-reduction Regimen," *Arthroscopy* 12 (December 23, 2007): 1320–25.
2. T. Krosshaug, A. Nakamae, B. P. Boden, et al., "Mechanisms of Anterior Cruciate Ligament Injury in Basketball: Video Analysis of 39 Cases," *American Journal of Sports Medicine* 35, no. 3 (2007): 359–66.
3. B. P. Boden, G. S. Dean, J. A. Feagin, et al., "Mechanisms of Anterior Cruciate Ligament Injury," *Orthopedics* 23, no. 6 (2000): 573–78.
4. M. Kritz, J. Cronin, and P. Hume, "The Bodyweight Squat: A Movement Screen for the Squat Pattern," *National Strength and Conditioning Association* 31, no. 1 (2009): 76–85.

Chapter 2
Barbell Squat Technique

2.1 Maintaining Postural Integrity
In the last chapter, we discussed how to teach the perfect bodyweight squat. We talked about a strategy to maintain stability during a bodyweight squat by holding our arms out in front of us. By doing this, it brings our lower back (lumbar spine) into a good neutral position.

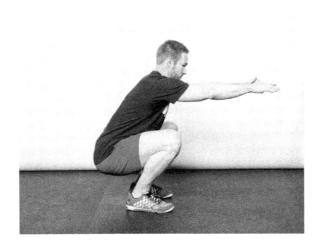

In order to maintain the integrity of our posture when we squat with a barbell, we need to adapt our technique. A barbell places higher demand on our body to stabilize our trunk. In order to meet these demands, we need to find a way to increase our stability. A stable core is the platform for which we can perform efficient, powerful movements.

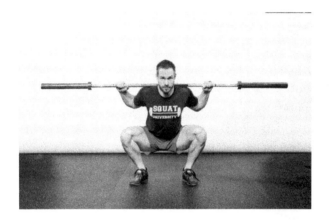

2.1.1 Core Stability

The quality of our movement during the squat is dictated by how stable we maintain our trunk. A bare spine, without any muscles, is nothing but a stack of bones. Without the continuous collaboration of the twenty-nine pairs of muscles that make up our trunk and the fascia that holds them together, the weight of our upper body alone would be enough to collapse our spine.[1]

Very often, we see athletes believe that they can improve trunk stability through exercises such as sit-ups or crunches. In reality, those movements build isolated muscular strength, not stability. There is a difference between strength and the ability to stabilize.

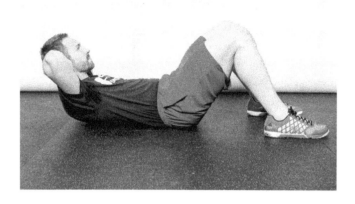

Strength is the ability to produce force. The harder you can push or pull a weight, the stronger your muscles are. Stability is the ability to resist movement at one part of your body while movement takes place around it. A stable spine resists being bent in two by the massive weight of the barbell.

Strengthening a stabilizer (such as the abdominal muscles with crunches or the low back erectors with endless hyperextensions) will not cause those muscles to necessarily stabilize more effectively. Core stability is the synchronous action of the abdominal muscles along with the muscles of the back, hip, pelvic girdle, and diaphragm and surrounding fascia. When working together, they keep the spine in a safe and stable position while we move. Therefore, core stability has nothing to do with how many crunches you perform or hypers off the glut-ham machine. The essence of stability is based on two things: timing and coordinated recruitment.

In order to recruit our core muscles prior to the squat, the cue to "brace for a punch" is recommended. This action increases the stability of our lower back and locks it into a good neutral position. When we turn on these muscles prior to the descent of the squat, we proactively prepare our body to handle the load that we are trying to carry.

2.1.2 Proper Breathing

It is not enough to only brace for a punch when we squat. If you want to move massive weights in a safe manner, you must also learn how to breathe properly. For too long, professionals in the strength and medical fields have failed to incorporate proper breathing during lifts. Many have essentially approached our core like a balloon, trying to strengthen the outside rubber walls instead of learning how to increase the pressure within.

Fitness and medical professionals are taught, "Breathe in on the way down and breathe out on the way up." This is fine for an exercise involving light weight and higher repetitions (i.e., bench press three sets of ten reps). This breathing mechanic, however, is not entirely recommended when performing the barbell squat. Can you imagine what would happen if a powerlifter let out his entire breath on the way up from squatting one thousand pounds?

When we squat heavy weight with a barbell (for example, anything over 80 percent of your one-rep maximum), it is advised to take a large breath and hold it through the entire repetition. Usually this type of breathing is not needed for higher repetition sets with low weight. However, when you are squatting heavy for a few reps, it is crucial. This breath should be taken prior to and in coordination with the cue to "brace for a punch." Doing so allows us to dramatically stabilize our core.

To learn how to properly breathe during the squat, try this simple test. Place one hand on your stomach and the other on your side (near your lower ribs). Now take a big breath. If you did this properly, you will feel your stomach rise and fall. You will also feel your lower rib cage expand laterally (out to the side). Essentially, you are feeling the volume increasing inside your core. When we take a big breath, the diaphragm just below our lungs contracts, and it will descend toward our stomach.[2]

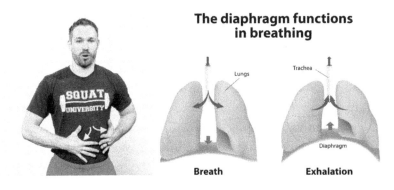

If you breathe improperly, you will instead notice the chest rise and fall. Breathing in this manner does little to increase the volume of our intra-abdominal cavity because the diaphragm is never fully utilized. So why is this rise in volume so important?

When we correctly breathe "into our stomach" and combine the action with bracing our core, we find that something special happens. With your hand on your stomach again, take a big breath one more time. After the breath is taken, brace your core muscles as if you are about to receive a Mike Tyson punch to the gut. Combining these actions increases the pressure inside the abdominal cavity (intra-abdominal pressure or IAP). This is because the volume can no longer expand. Increased IAP has been shown in research to be the most effective method to stabilize your lower back during barbell training.[3, 4]

This must be done in a step-by-step manner. If we brace first and then try to take a big breath, we limit how much pressure we can create.

This is because the diaphragm cannot fully contract and descend if the core is already maximally braced. Increasing IAP in this manner helps stabilize the lower spine to an even greater degree than with bracing alone.[5]

To experience the connection between the pressure in your core and your overall strength, try this simple test. Put a barbell on your back and exhale all of the air from your lungs. Feel for how the bar feels on your back. Next, take a big breath and brace your core. Try to create pressure in a 360-degree manner around your core as if wearing a tight corset. Remember, the breath must be taken to expand the front, side, and back of your core. Do you notice anything different?

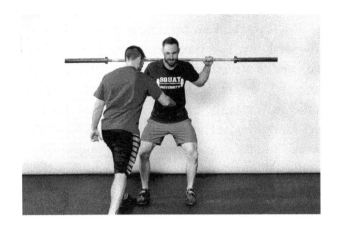

The weight of the bar should now feel much lighter on your back. Does it make sense that using this maneuver might have some application to lifting heavy weights in the squat? This is how the strongest weightlifters and powerlifters are able to squat tremendous weights without breaking in half.

Holding this breath during the execution of the squat will often cause a forced grunt on the ascent. This happens when we try to limit the natural desire to exhale on the way up. This forced hold is called the Valsalva maneuver. Limiting our breath from escaping in this powerful manner is essential in order to maintain our spinal stability.

To perform the Valsalva maneuver correctly, the breath is exhaled forcefully against a closed airway. This is where the saying "inhale on the way down and exhale on the way up" takes a turn. Exhaling a breath completely during the ascent of a squat can lead to a severe drop in IAP.

As the pressure in our abdomen drops, the stability of the spine will decrease. It doesn't matter how hard you brace your core muscles. If you let your breath out completely, you will instantly lose stability. This transfers harmful pressures onto the small, vulnerable structures of the spine (intervertebral discs and ligaments). This is like letting the air out of a balloon too fast. As the air leaves the balloon, it becomes less stable. The same goes for our body. However, if we only let a small amount of air escape the balloon by maintaining our squeeze on the opening, the balloon stays stable for longer.

In order to keep the pressure in our abdomen and our spinal stability intact, the exhale must be forcefully stopped from fully escaping. Essentially, we need to keep our fingers on the opening of the balloon. There are different ways to do this. Some lifters will use a grunting method or a "tss" sound as they slowly exhale through a small hole in their lips. Both of these methods allow the pressure in the abdomen to stay at a high level during the entirety of the lift.

The breath should never be held for more than a few seconds during the squat. Doing so can dramatically increase blood pressure and cause blackouts and other cardiovascular injury for those at risk. While the Valsalva maneuver (even when held for short periods) has been shown to cause an increase in systolic blood pressure, it is very safe for healthy athletes. For most, this temporary rise in blood pressure is not harmful. That being said, older individuals and anyone with a history of heart disease should use it with caution.[6]

Take Away
A proper squat is all about maintaining proper spinal stability. When we combine the coordinated bracing ability of our core muscles and harness the power of our breath, we allow our body to move properly and lift tremendous weights safely.

2.2 The High-Bar Back Squat

The high-bar back squat is typically one of the first barbell exercises young athletes are taught today. By perfecting technique, an athlete has the potential to lift bigger weights with less risk for injury.

It doesn't matter how hard you push. It doesn't matter how well the training plan is written. Any flaws in technique will limit your maximum potential.

The Lift Off

The first part of successful barbell squats is at the rack. The bar should be set around chest height. Setting the bar too high or too low can force lifters to put themselves in a dangerous position in order to unrack and rerack the weighted barbell.

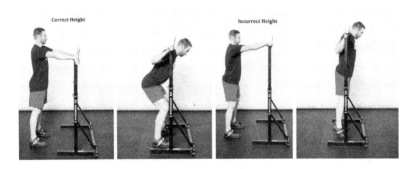

The next step is to get the bar into the correct position on your back. Pull yourself under the bar and trap it tightly against the tops of your shoulders and back of your neck. By pulling your shoulder blades together, a "shelf" will appear through the contraction of the upper back muscles. The bar should be positioned on top of this shelf.

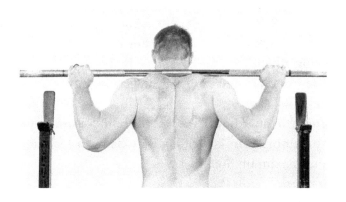

The type of grip taken on the bar will be a personal choice. Some will hook their thumb under the bar while others will keep it on top of the bar (monkey grip). Regardless of the way you decide to grip the bar, a neutral wrist alignment is ideal. The straightforward wrist allows the weight of the bar to be safely secured on the back without placing too much pressure on the elbows.

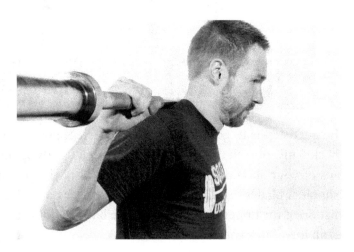

It's now time to unrack the bar. Position yourself under the bar with your feet evenly spaced around shoulder width. Take a big breath while bracing your core. Extend your hips and knees at the same time (with even pressure between both legs) and stand up with the bar.

Often athletes try to unrack the bar with their feet staggered. With lighter weight on the barbell, it is easy to get away with this move. However, as soon as the weight increases to high levels, unracking the barbell in this manner can be dangerous.

It is also common to see athletes try to unrack the bar without a braced core. Without bracing your core, it's difficult to organize and create appropriate stability needed to complete the lift. Case in point: you don't see many nine-hundred-pound squats where the athlete unracks the weight in a casual manner. The tremendous weight of the bar would instantly crush the athlete.

<u>The Descent</u>

The descent of the barbell squat follows the same principles of the bodyweight squat with two small changes: foot placement and breathing mechanics. Now that an athlete is squatting with a barbell, he or she may turn his or her toes out slightly. This allows some athletes to squat deeper while maintaining stability.

After unracking the bar properly, take three slow steps backward and establish your squat stance. The width of this stance should be comfortable and allow for full range of motion. For this reason, every athlete will have a slight difference in stance width.

Next, the tripod foot needs to be engaged. All three points of the foot need to be in equal contact with the ground. If done properly, the foot will move into a full arched position. This allows the foot to remain stable and support the rest of the body just like the base layer for a house of cards.

The next step is to create external rotation torque at the hips. By squeezing your glutes, torque is generated at the hip joint and the knees are brought into correct alignment with the toes.

Some coaches will use the cue to "drive the knees wide." This cue works great for a number of athletes, especially those whose knees collapse inward during the squat. For others, it can lead the athlete to become unbalanced. Therefore, it must be used on an individual basis. Driving the knees too far to the outside can cause the foot to turn on its side. This is like a tripod trying to remain in balance on only two of the three points. Whatever cue you use, make sure the entire foot stays in contact with the ground and the knee tracks in line with the toes.

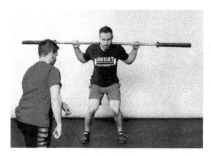 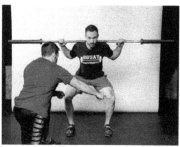

Next, take another big breath "into your stomach" and brace your core as if Mike Tyson is going to punch you. The last step is to engage the posterior chain (glutes and hamstrings). This happens with a proper hip hinge. Push your hips backward slightly and bring your chest forward. During a high-bar squat, this hip engagement will be fairly small. If the hips move back too far, the chest will reflexively drop forward. This will leave you off balance. Once the hips are engaged slightly and your body is in balance, start your squat by sitting your butt straight down on your heels. Don't think about going to a certain depth. Just squat.

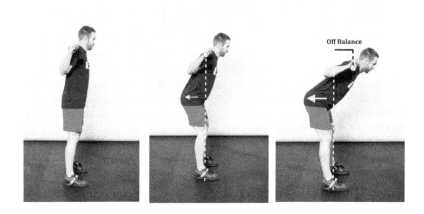

The Bottom Position

In order to produce efficient strength and power during the squat, we must remain balanced. This requires our center of gravity to stay directly over the middle of our feet. During the bodyweight squat, our center of gravity is located near the middle of our stomach. Depending on the physical makeup of an athlete (height, weight, leg length, etc.), this location may change slightly.

In order to stay balanced during the bodyweight squat, the torso has to be inclined over the knees. During the barbell squat, however, the bar now becomes our center of gravity. Due to the position of the weight during the high-bar back squat, a more upright torso position will be used.

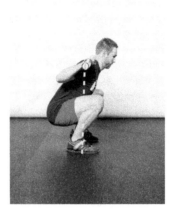

This technique change will cause the knees to eventually move forward past the toes in order to reach full depth. This shift balances the load between the quads and glutes. It also requires an athlete to have adequate ankle mobility. For this reason, athletes with stiff ankles can often show perfect squat technique with no weight but will struggle during the high-bar variation.

The high-bar back squat is usually performed to a greater depth than the low-bar version (commonly used by powerlifters). In the competitive sport of weightlifting (i.e., snatch and clean and jerk), the weight is often caught in a very deep squat. The high-bar technique therefore translates well into the sport of weightlifting and CrossFit.

That being said, not all athletes are training to compete in the sport of weightlifting. For this reason, the barbell squat does not always need to be taken ass-to-grass. Depth of a barbell squat will be specific to the demands of the sport an athlete participates in. Every athlete should be able to hit at least parallel depth. This means the crease of the hip will be parallel with the tops of the knee.

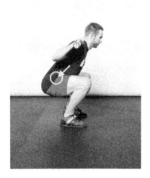 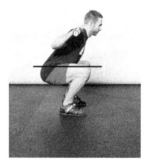

The Ascent

The ascent of the squat is all about staying balanced. From the bottom of the squat, the hips and chest should rise at the same rate.

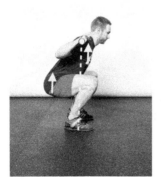 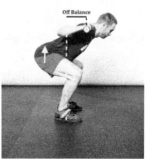

Elite weightlifters at times will use a forceful transition in their bottom position. This is a skilled maneuver that can allow an athlete to lift more weight. Technique is imperative if this powerful move is to be attempted. Alignment of the knees must be maintained. If performed correctly, the rebound will feel like a spring releasing, propelling you upward with tremendous power.

The torso must also be maintained in a stable position during this part of the lift. Often inexperienced athletes will let their back collapse and round forward. If an athlete tries to forcefully bounce out of the bottom position without proper control, he or she risks losing stability at the low back. When this happens, harmful forces are instantly placed on the vulnerable structures of the back.

A forceful transition should always be learned under the direct supervision of an experienced coach. If performed incorrectly, it can easily lead to technique breakdown and eventual injury.

High-Bar Sequence

1. Pin the barbell tightly against the shelf of your upper back.
2. Establish a stable tripod foot.
3. Generate external rotation torque at the hips. (Verbal cue: squeeze your glutes.)
4. Create a rigid trunk by taking a big breath and holding it tight. (Verbal cue: big breath and core tight.)
5. Hip hinge to engage the posterior chain. (Verbal cue: hips back.)

6. Remain balanced by keeping the bar over the midfoot during the entire squat.
7. Hips and chest rise at the same rate on the ascent. (Verbal cue: drive the hips up and chest up.)

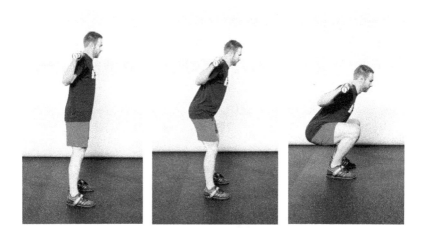

2.3 The Low-Bar Back Squat

It is now time to talk about the low-bar back squat. Athletes competing in the sport of powerlifting typically use this variation as it allows them to lift more weight.

The Liftoff

Taking the barbell out of the rack correctly is the first step to any successful squat. Just like the high-bar back squat and front squat, the bar should be set at around chest height. A general rule of thumb is to set the bar lower instead of higher. The worst situation is when you have to tip toe up just to get the bar on and off.

Next, we need to position the barbell correctly on the back. Pull yourself under the bar and trap it tightly against the back of your shoulders. By pulling your shoulder blades together, a "shelf" will appear through the contraction of the midback muscles. The barbell should be positioned on this shelf. This will end up being two to three inches lower than where the bar is held during the high-bar back squat. If you have never done the low-bar back squat, this may feel uncomfortable and unusual.

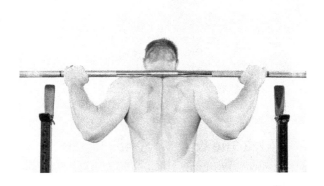

The width of the grip you use on the barbell should be based on comfort. Most powerlifters are seen using a wide grip on the bar (around the notches). However, this isn't an absolute that everyone must follow. Taking a standard grip on the barbell (just outside shoulder width) can be used with a low-bar squat. That being said, you must have sufficient upper-body mobility to do so. Taking too narrow of a grip when you are lacking flexibility in the chest/shoulders can lead to increased stress on the elbow joint.

It's now time to unrack the bar. Position yourself under the bar with your feet evenly spaced (around shoulder width apart). Take a big breath while bracing your core.

Once you are ready, lift the bar off the rack by driving upward with your hips. Take a few short steps backward out of the rack. *Always step back out of the rack.* Stepping forward means you must rerack the weight after your set by going backward. This can be very dangerous (especially if you are fatigued and lifting heavy weight), as you will not be able to clearly see the rack hooks to safely set the bar down.

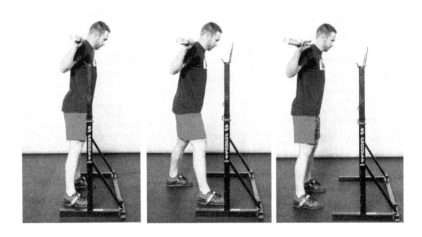

Once the weight on your back comes to a rest, it's time to establish a solid foundation for your squat. Always ensure you're in complete control of your body and the weight has stopped moving. Now you are ready to squat.

The Descent
The stance you take during any squat should allow you to remain balanced and reach full depth. Athletes who compete in powerlifting will often use a wider stance when using the low-bar technique. The degree of toe-out angle will vary based on an individual's anatomy and mobility. A general recommendation is to point the toes out slightly (between ten to twenty degrees).

The next step is to squeeze your glutes and drive your knees in line with your feet. Take another big breath into your stomach and brace your core as if you're going to receive a punch to the stomach. The last step is to engage the posterior chain (glutes and hamstrings). Push your hips backward and bring your chest forward. Once the hips are engaged, start your squat. Always descend in a controlled manner. Don't think about stopping at a certain depth. Just squat.

The Bottom Position
While no two squats will look exactly the same, you still have to line the bar over the middle of the foot (this is an absolute of squatting). To keep the bar (which is now positioned lower on the back) centered over the midfoot, the chest is going to be inclined over the knees more so than the other squat techniques. Depending on the physical makeup of an athlete (height, weight, leg length, etc.), the amount of trunk inclination is going to vary. Some athletes will have a more upright torso while others will be very inclined.

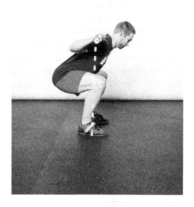

In the book *Starting Strength*, Mark Rippetoe explains that most balance problems in the low-bar squat are usually due to a back angle that is too vertical.[6] If you feel off balance with your squat, make sure you are sitting your hips back enough and allowing your chest to lean forward.

The bottom position of this squat will not require the knees to move forward too much. The low-bar squat inherently places more of the load on the posterior chain (hamstrings and glutes) when compared to the front squat and high-bar squat.

You don't need to have amazing ankle mobility to perfect the low-bar squat, which is why powerlifters will often wear a flat-sole shoe like the classic Chuck Taylors compared to a weightlifting shoe with a raised heel.

The Ascent

The ascent of the squat is all about hip drive. From the bottom of the squat, the hips should be driven straight up. In order to keep the bar from tracking toward the toes, make sure to also drive the chest up at the same time. Failure to do so will cause the hips to rise excessively and the torso to remain forward. Doing so will often cause the bar to track toward the toes. This position places harmful forces on the lower back and can easily lead to injury.

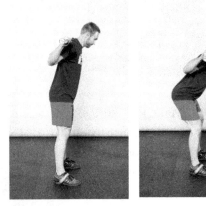
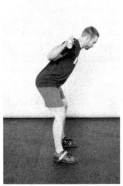
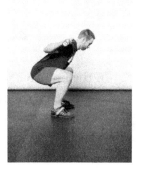

Low-Bar Sequence

1. Pin the barbell tightly against the shelf of your midback, just below your shoulder muscles (posterior deltoids).
2. Establish a stable tripod foot.
3. Generate external rotation torque at the hips. (Verbal cue: squeeze your glutes.)
4. Create a rigid trunk by taking a big breath and holding it tight. (Verbal cue: big breath and core tight.)

5. Hip hinge to engage the posterior chain. (Verbal cue: hips back.)
6. Remain balanced by keeping the bar over the midfoot during the entire squat.
7. Use hip drive to stand up from the bottom position. (Verbal cue: drive the hips and chest up.)

2.4 The Front Squat

While the back squat is often labeled as the "king of all exercises," the front squat usually follows close behind. Like many of the other barbell lifts, it is often performed incorrectly.

The Lift Off

The first step in performing a perfect front squat begins at the rack. To start, the bar needs to be set at shoulder height. Inexperienced athletes will often place the bar too high in the rack. This requires the athlete to overextend in order to unrack the bar. While many can get away with this early on, it can be dangerous when attempting to squat a heavy weight.

The next step is to position the bar properly on your chest. Start by gripping the bar at shoulder width. For weightlifters and CrossFitters, this is the same grip used to perform the barbell-clean movement. From this position, pull yourself under the bar while at the same time pushing your chest through the ceiling. The elbows should be lifted together to the highest possible position.

If done correctly, this will create a shelf for the bar to sit comfortably on top of the shoulders and chest. Doing so will also increase the rigidity of your upper back. This will help you maintain an upright trunk position throughout the entire lift. Leaving the elbows in low position can lead to a rounded upper back. This greatly increases the odds of dropping the weight as it gets heavy. You will also place your body at risk for injury.

Mobility issues at the shoulder and/or thoracic spine (upper back) may cause the lifter to not be able to reach the high elbow position. It's acceptable to leave the fingers in contact with the bar and have an open palm to reach the high elbow position.

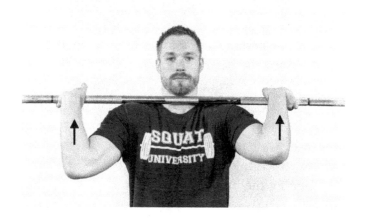

This allows the weight to stay balanced on top of the shoulders. Athletes who are new to the front squat will often try to maintain a grip on the bar when they don't have the appropriate mobility. Over time, this can place unwanted stress on the wrists and elbows. It can also lead to pain and eventual injury when attempting to lift heavy weight.

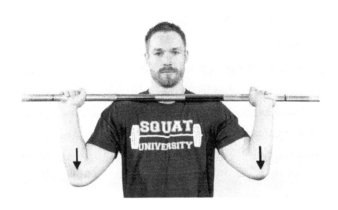

It's now time to unrack the barbell. Position yourself under the bar with your feet evenly spaced around shoulder width. Take a big breath while bracing your core. Extend your hips and knees at the same time (with even pressure between both legs) and stand up with the bar.

Filling your lungs with air and bracing your core before you lift the barbell out of the rack is essential, especially when attempting to squat heavy weight. This big breath and bracing technique can make the heavy weight feel lighter when the bar is on your chest. Stabilizing the core with a big breath will allow you to lift massive weights without breaking in half.

Just like the high-bar back squat, the front squat will also use a straightforward or slightly upward eye gaze. This will keep harmful forces from being placed on your neck during the lift.

The Descent
With the bar secured properly on your shoulders, take three steps backward in a slow and steady manner. Set your feet in a

comfortable and stable position. Foot placement should mimic the same position used during the high-bar back squat. The feet may be pointed slightly outward and the stance should be at a comfortable width. Each athlete will have a slightly different stance width based on his or her individual anatomy and level of mobility.

Prior to initiating the descent of the squat, establish a proper foundation with your feet. Next, squeeze the glutes in order to bring your knees into good alignment with the toes. Stabilize your back by taking a breath "into the stomach" and bracing the core muscles.

In order to perform a proper hip hinge during the front squat, the hips will push back very slightly. This allows you to engage the powerhouse of your body (the glutes of the posterior chain). By hinging the hips back slightly, the bar also remains over the midfoot. This allows the body to remain in balance. The amount of backward movement will be even less than the high-bar back squat.

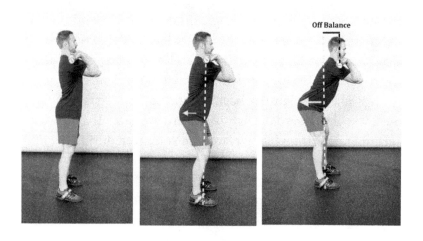

It's a misconception that with the front squat, the knees need to move first. This misconception will lead the athlete to potentially overload the knee joint, become off balance, and capsize his or her potential to lift heavy weight. The knees will still bend during this hip engagement. However, they should not push forward off the start.

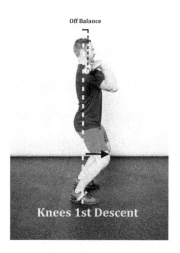

The Bottom Position

The bottom position of the front squat will closely mimic that of the high-bar back squat. The torso will remain fairly vertical in order to keep the bar on the shoulders.

The depth of the front squat will be based on the specific requirements of an athlete's sport choice and goals. An athlete competing in football or baseball, for example, will only need to descend to a parallel position. This means the hip crease will be parallel to the knee joint.

For those training in the sport of weightlifting or competitive CrossFit, the hips should descend to the greatest depth possible. This will allow these athletes to develop the strength needed to meet the demands of their chosen sport where the clean and snatch are often taken in a deep-squat position.

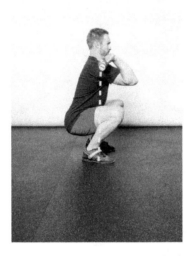

This deep-squat position will eventually cause the knees to translate forward over the toes. As we have discussed in prior articles, the body can handle the stresses of this forward knee position as long as two requirements are met. First, the knees must not move forward prematurely into this position. Second, proper training programming must be used to allow for proper recovery. **We need to be more concerned with *when* the knees move forward in the squat and not *if*.**

The Ascent

Once we have established a stable bottom position, it is time to begin the ascent. The ascent is all about keeping the torso in a good upright position. Often inexperienced athletes will let their back go round during this portion of the lift.

Often coaches will use the cue to keep the elbows up during the ascent. This can be a good cue to a point. We also need to cue athletes to drive their chest upward. A good front squat requires both high elbows and an upright trunk. Failing to cue both can lead to a rounded upper back and eventual injury.

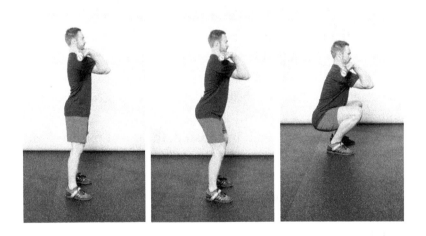

Front Squat Sequence

1. Position the bar securely on your chest and shoulders with your elbows high.
2. Establish a stable tripod foot.

3. Generate external rotation torque at the hips. (Verbal cue: squeeze your glutes.)
4. Create a rigid trunk by taking a big breath and holding it tight. (Verbal cue: big breath and core tight.)
5. Slightly hip hinge to engage the posterior chain. Keep the trunk in a vertical position. (Verbal cue: push the hips back only a bit.)
6. Remain balanced by keeping the bar over the midfoot during the entire squat.
7. Maintain an upright chest position with the elbows raised high. (Verbal cue: drive the chest straight up.)

2.5 The Overhead Squat

Prior to the turn of the century, the overhead squat was primarily used by competitive weightlifters. Olympic weightlifting coaches use the overhead squat as a teaching progression for novice athletes. The overhead squat is used to strengthen the bottom position of a barbell snatch.

Since the recent boom in CrossFit, the use of the overhead squat has become more widespread. It has been transformed into a staple exercise for training for many sports and has even been used in competition.

In order to perform this lift correctly, an athlete must have a high level of coordination, balance, and mobility.

Bar or PVC Pipe?

For inexperienced athletes or young children first learning to overhead squat, a barbell may be too heavy. For this reason, a lightweight PVC pipe or a broomstick can be used in place.

To find a proper grip with a PVC pipe that has no markings, try this simple method. Stand tall and pull your elbows out to the side. Your arms should end up in a ninety-degree *L* position. Measure the distance between your right and left hands. Now mark that distance on the PVC pipe. Place your index finger on this line when grasping the pipe during the overhead squat.

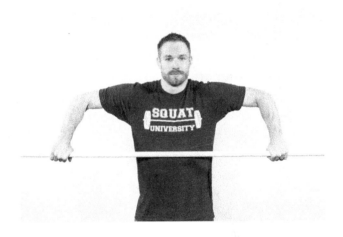

When transitioning to the bar, athletes will usually take their grip a few inches from the end of the bar. This will be the same grip taken for the barbell snatch lift. Athletes with longer arms may need to take a grip almost to the end of the barbell, near the collars. Those with shorter arms may only need to place their grip around the outer notch of the bar.

The Setup
To start, hold the barbell on your upper back. This will be the same starting position as the high-bar back squat. After

unracking the barbell properly, you will need to hoist the weight to the overhead position. This can be done in a number of ways depending on the amount of weight on the barbell and the individual preference of the lifter.

When an athlete is first learning how to perform the overhead squat, most coaches will teach a simple push-press to hoist the barbell to the overhead position. Once the weight increases to a significant load, a push-jerk or split-jerk is recommended for experienced weightlifters.

To start the push-press, pull your elbows underneath the bar. This will place your arms in an efficient position to drive the barbell upward. The hands should be at a snatch-grip width.

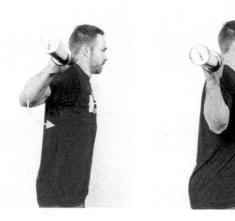

Next, take and hold a large breath. Brace your core muscles as if about to receive a punch to the stomach. The dip-and-drive movement is then used to push the barbell overhead.

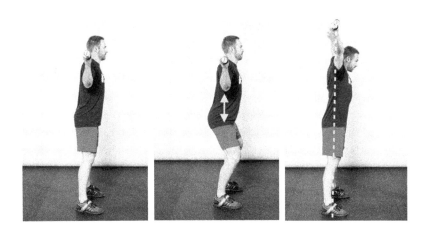

Drop your hips straight down a few inches while keeping your torso in a vertical position. A cue that is often used to maintain this straight dip is to imagine the feeling of your back sliding down a wall. If the hips drive backward during the dip, it will cause the chest to push forward. This will set you up to push the barbell forward into a bad overhead position.

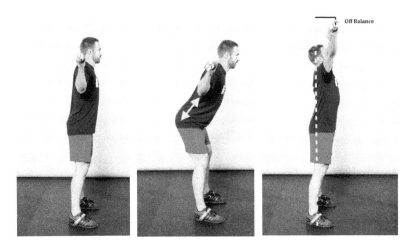

During the controlled dip, the knees should be kept in proper alignment with the feet. This will allow for an efficient transfer of power from the legs to the arms during the push. If the knees collapse inward on the dip, you will limit the potential upward driving power you can create with your legs.

After the dip is performed, push the barbell straight up by extending the hips, knees, and ankles in a powerful motion. The barbell should end up in a stable overhead position just over the back of your neck.

Your head can be pushed forward slightly to allow for this stable position. Be careful not to push the head too far forward. This will cause the chest to lean forward excessively and throw you off balance.

To keep the barbell overhead in a firm position, the elbows should be completely locked out. You will have a difficult time keeping the barbell from wavering around if the elbows are not completely straight.

In this overhead position, the barbell should rest in the center of the palm. The wrists should be slightly extended. This is a position of stability that will not cause too much stress to the wrist joint. Do *not* try to keep a neutral straight wrist during an overhead squat.

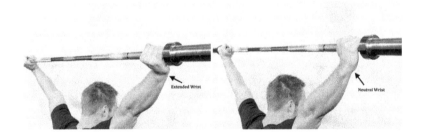

Make sure to gaze straight forward or slightly upward. This will place the neck in a neutral position and limit any unwanted stresses. Looking upward excessively or down toward your feet can throw you off balance.

The Descent
Once you have stabilized the bar overhead, it's time to start the descent. Push your hips back slightly to engage the posterior chain. As you begin your squat, think about sitting your hips onto your heels. This cue helps limit a large hip hinge that can throw you off balance. Control the descent to full depth.

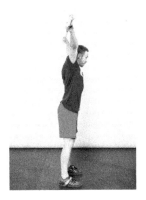
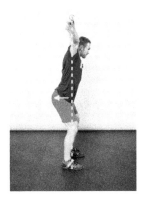

The bar should always remain aligned over the middle of your foot for balance and stability. Proper technique is critical, as a missed lift can lead to injury. If at any time the lift becomes unstable, push the bar forward or backward and dump the bar to the ground. Both are completely safe alternatives for missing a weight. I recommend using bumper plates whenever doing overhead squats. Be aware of your surroundings.

The Bottom Position

The knees should be allowed to translate forward over the toes at the deepest part of this squat. This will allow you to maintain the desired vertical trunk position to keep the bar overhead.

The Ascent

The hips and chest should rise at the same rate during the ascent of the squat. If the hips rise fast and the chest stays forward, the barbell will drift toward your toes, likely causing you to drop the weight.

Once you've come to a stable standing position, slowly control the bar down to the shelf position on your upper back. Letting the bar drop too quickly can lead to serious injury to the neck. If the weight is heavy, a slight dip can lessen the intensity of receiving the bar.

Overhead Squat Sequence

1. Establish a safe starting position. The barbell should be resting on the upper traps (as with the high-bar back squat) with the elbows pulled under the barbell.
2. Create a rigid trunk by taking a big breath and holding it tight. (Verbal cue: big breath and core tight.)
3. Use a controlled dip and drive to push the bar into an overhead position. (Verbal cue: slide your back down a wall and drive upward with power.)
4. Stabilize the barbell. (Verbal cue: drive your hands to the ceiling and lock your elbows out.)
5. Use a slight hip hinge to engage the posterior chain.

THE SQUAT BIBLE

6. Remain balanced by keeping the bar positioned over the midfoot the entire squat.
7. Hips and chest rise at the same rate on the ascent.

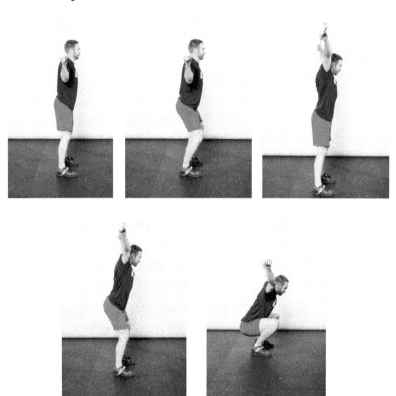

Notes

1. J. J. Crisco, M. M. Panjabi, I. Yamamoto, and T. R. Oxland, "Stability of the Human Ligamentous Lumbar Spine. Part II: Experiment," *Clinical Biomechanics* 7 (1992): 27–32.
2. P. Kolar, J. Neuwirth, J. Sanda, et al., "Analysis of Diaphragm Movement during Tidal Breathing and during Its Activation while Breath Holding Using MRI Synchronized Spirometry," *Physiological Research* 58 (2009): 383–92.
3. D. A. Hackett and C-M. Chow, "The Valsalva Maneuver: Its Effect on Intra-abdominal Pressure and Safety Issues During Resistance Exercise," *Journal of Strength and Conditioning Research* 27, no. 8 (2013): 2338–45.
4. S. G. Grenier and S. M. McGill, "Quantification of Lumbar Stability by Using 2 Different Abdominal Activation Strategies," *Archives of Physical Medicine and Rehabilitation* 88, no. 1 (2007): 54–62.
5. J. Cholewicki, K. Juluru, and S. M. McGill, "Intra-abdominal Pressure Mechanism for Stabilizing the Lumbar Spine," *Journal of Biomechanics* 32, no. 1 (1999): 13–17.
6. M. Rippetoe, *Starting Strength: Basic Barbell Training*, 3rd ed. (Wichita Falls, TX: The Aasgaard Company, 2011).

Photo Attribution

1. The Diaphragm: Designua/Shutterstock.com

Chapter 3
The Joint-by-Joint Concept

In this chapter, we're going to talk about one of the most thought-provoking and influential approaches to understanding the human body: the joint-by-joint concept. Now, before we start, I want to make it known that this concept is not new or of my own creation. Physical therapist Gray Cook and strength coach Mike Boyle shaped this concept based on their observations and history working with athletes. They have written extensively on it in the past, and I definitely recommend checking out their expanded writings on the topic.

Their simple and straightforward concept is a game changer when it comes to how we as coaches, medical practitioners, and athletes view the human body. This philosophy has influenced the way I approach and treat my athletes as a doctor of physical therapy. The joint-by-joint concept is an idea I would like to share with you. We will also discuss how it relates to the squat.

Human movement is extremely complex. It is so complex that it lends itself to the illustration of a symphony orchestra composed of hundreds of simultaneous and intricate muscle actions. Some muscles create movement while others stabilize and hinder movement. Just as an orchestra changes tempo and shapes its sound in a united manner, our body must move and flow in a united manner as well.

Each joint in the body tends to have a specific function and purpose that is required for efficient movement to take place. In this stacked series of joints emerges a tendency for alternating series of mobile joints moving on top of stable joints. With an appreciation of what each joint requires, we can then "connect the dots" in our understanding of how the body works together to produce efficient movement.

First let's define two terms that describe the way our body functions.

- Mobility: describes the ability of the joint complex to move freely in an unrestricted manner through full range of motion. In basic terminology, this is our ability to move at a certain segment.
- Stability: describes the ability of a joint complex to maintain position while motion takes place somewhere else. This is simply the ability to control the motion at a certain segment. Stability can also be synonymous with the term *motor control*.

Let's look at a simple breakdown of the primary needs associated with each joint in the joint-by-joint concept.

- Foot = Stability
- Ankle = Mobility
- Knee = Stability
- Hip = Mobility

- Lumbar Spine = Stability
- Thoracic Spine = Mobility
- Scapula = Stability
- Shoulder = Mobility

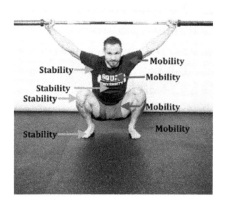

These labels are based off of common tendencies, patterns, and problems that we as practitioners have found over time. What we see is that athletes who develop injuries have similar mobility and stability problems. The overwhelming consensus in practical experience shows us that when the body is unable to adequately demonstrate mobility and stability at certain parts of the body, movement breakdown occurs and injury ensues. Let me explain.

- <u>The foot</u> is an area of the body that could benefit from increased stability and motor control due to its tendency to become unstable during movement. A recent article published in the *British Journal of Sports Medicine* compared the stability our "core" provides to our lower back to the role of the smaller muscles of our foot that work to maintain the same type of motor control during movement.[1] This control inevitably creates the stability of the foot for which all human movement such as squatting is based upon. While proper shoe wear does play an important part in the performance and injury processes, there is no denying we could all benefit from increased stability of the foot. When the foot has a stability problem, it will directly affect the ankle joint.

- The ankle is an area of the body that would benefit from increased mobility and flexibility. Inherently, we see many athletic injuries that occur when the ankle develops stiffness and loses flexibility—particularly in the movement of dorsiflexion (the movement of the knee forward over the toe during the deepest portion of the squat). The tendency for the ankle joint complex to become immobile then affects the role of the joint directly above (the knee) and the area below (the foot).
- The knee joint is an area of the body that would benefit from increased stability. Obviously, the knee needs to be mobile when we squat in order to reach a solid bottom position. Unfortunately, the problem we see is that athletes who develop pain tend to have unstable knees, especially when they squat. When we squat, jump, run, and cut, we need to be able to control the knee. The knee must stay in proper alignment (stability) to avoid

injury. Many injuries occur because the knee tends to bow in instead of staying aligned over the foot.
- The hip joint is an area of the body that shows a tendency to benefit from increased mobility due to its tendency to become immobile and stiff. If the hip loses its mobility, it will affect the role of the joint complex directly above (the lower back) and below (the knee). What we've come to find is that the all-too-common "lower back pain" is caused by a lack of hip mobility.[2] For this reason, it wouldn't matter how much strength and stability work you perform on the core—if the hip mobility is never addressed, no change in pain will occur.
- The lower back (lumbar spine) is a joint complex that requires stability. Very often, we see that the lower back loses stability. When this happens, our body develops compensations that lead to stiffness, decreased power production, and eventual pain. When looking at squats, a stable lower back is a necessity; otherwise, you risk injury. Food for thought: Ensuring this stability is more than just performing planks and endless sit-ups. Strength is not the same as stability. A strong core and stable spine prevent excessive movement.
- The mid to upper back (thoracic spine) is a joint complex that requires mobility. This area of the body is inherently very stable due to the support it helps create with the ribs for our vital organs. However, we all could benefit from increasing our available mobility and flexibility to this region. For most people, the thoracic spine stiffens due to excessive sitting all day at work and

playing on the computer and smart phone. The majority of Americans have crappy posture. Crappy posture limits ability to perform high-level movements, such as the overhead squat and snatch/jerk. Not to mention that poor posture/inflexible thoracic spine raises the risk of shoulder impingements and other shoulder injuries.

The process goes on and on up the body, in a simple alternating pattern. Stable joints stacked on top of mobile joints. When a mobile joint becomes immobile, the stable joint above or below will give up its stability and move as compensation. This is how injury occurs in our body. The simple format of the joint-by-joint approach allows us to understand the body to a deeper extent.

Recently, we have seen a substantial shift in the way athletes are trained and rehabilitated after injury. In the past, the paradigm of training and rehabilitation was to concentrate solely on one part of the body. We essentially viewed the body through a microscope. Fueled by the golden era of bodybuilding and the desire to look like Arnold Schwarzenegger, athletes would enter a workout to train their "back and biceps" or "chest and triceps." This mindset was predicated in the thought process that a stronger and bigger muscle would lead to increased performance. Athletes who injured their back would go to a physical therapist and perform hours of core work while lying on a bed. Rarely would a therapist make the connection that limited ankle mobility could have a potential connection to the lack in core stability. However, eventually a more intelligent approach to the athlete started to appear. The mantra "train movements not muscles" started to penetrate throughout the sport training and rehabilitation world.

Today athletes enter a training session to work on explosive movement through the power clean and back squat. A physical therapist will now spend a large majority of the time helping an injured patient with back pain recover through teaching core stability principles over a variety of movement patterns such as the squat or lunge. We now have the connection to realize that in order to address an injured area of the body, we need to also assess the joint above and below the site of pain. We as a society are starting to see that the missing link between optimal performance and injury is in the way we move as a whole. We are finally putting away the microscope and looking through the looking glass of movement.

Recently, I was working with a CrossFit athlete who was complaining of knee pain—one of the most common injuries to an athlete in any sport. She could run without pain. She could jump rope without pain. However, she could not squat with a barbell, snatch, or perform pistol squats without pain.

During our first meeting, I asked her to perform two simple bodyweight movements—a deep bodyweight squat and a pistol squat to full depth. Instantly, I observed a theoretical "crack" in her movement foundation. Simply put, she could not squat with good technique. During her bodyweight squat, she turned her toes out excessively and allowed her knees to roll in slightly at the bottom position. Her pistol squat was even worse as she was unable to even pass a parallel hip depth position without her knee collapsing inward.

Straight off the bat, this athlete had a movement issue that was causing her pain. By applying the joint-by-joint concept to this broken movement pattern, we were able to uncover a few problems that were all connected.

- Stiff ankles
- Unstable knees
- Immobile hips

The combination of these deficits led to knee pain. The most important aspect of the joint-by-joint approach is that it allows us to expand our view of how we approach the body. Given this CrossFit athlete had knee pain, many coaches and trainers may approach this injury by focusing solely on the knee itself. The doctor would hand out some pain medication and tell her to rest. Next, a therapist would prescribe a barrage of foam rolling, stretching, and icing the knee. Does this sound familiar to you?

Even if we acknowledged that there was an instability issue at the knee and started some stability training, the effects would be short lived. The stability we would create wouldn't be real whenever she needed to squat, clean, or snatch again. Until the immobility of the ankles and hips are addressed (the joints directly above and below), the knee will never fully stabilize in real-world situations. In his book *Movement*, Gray Cook wrote, "It's not about finding what came first, the chicken or the egg—you have to catch both or you can't manage either."

Let's return to our analogy from the start of this chapter. Movement in the body is synonymous with a skilled orchestra with dozens of musicians playing in a coordinated and synchronous fashion. Our usual response to pain is like telling the violins to stop playing because they sound bad. The pain, just like the poor-sounding instruments, is our warning that something isn't working correctly. Taking pain medication and placing ice on the knee because it hurts before ever examining the hip and ankle is just like silencing a section of the orchestra that is playing out of tune. In the end, you didn't fix the issue. The musicians' instruments are still out of tune. You just covered it up and stopped their playing for the time being.

By acknowledging that each joint complex has its own specific role, we can use a systematic approach to understanding how movement breaks down and injuries occur. In doing so, we can rid ourselves of pain but also maximize our potential to move and perform at the highest level possible. I challenge you to look at the big picture. When dealing with pain, look at the joint above and below. You may be surprised by what you find.

Notes

1. P. O. McKeon, J. Hertel, D. Bramble, and I. Davi, "The Foot Core System: A New Paradigm for Understanding Intrinsic Foot Muscle Function," *British Journal of Sports Medicine* 49 (2015): 290.
2. S. M. Roach, J. G. San Juan, D. N. Suprak, et al., "Passive Hip Range of Motion Is Reduced in Active Subjects with Chronic Low Back Pain Compared to Controls," *International Journal of Sports Physical Therapy* 10, no. 1 (February 2015): 13–20.

Chapter 4
The Stable Foot

In this chapter, we're going to cover a topic that is a little less understood by most. We are going to talk about your feet. Our feet set the foundation for every single functional movement. They provide a stable platform for the rest of our body to move.

Very often I find that athletes do not use their feet properly. Many coaches and physical therapists lose sight of how important the feet are when it comes to movement. Whether we are squatting, lunging, running, or jumping, a stable foot provides a platform for efficient and powerful movement for the rest of the body.

For this reason, it is important to establish a simple baseline for understanding our feet. The first thing we need to establish is that the foot is naturally mobile. There are over twenty-five bones spread across four different joints in the foot. This allows for a ton of movement. The role of our muscles therefore should be that of stability. The second we brace our bodies to lift that heavy barbell from the rack, we want our mobile foot to be instantaneously stable.

When we squat, we need the foot to be stable and maintain its natural arch. When we look at the main arch of our foot, we notice that it moves in relation to the rest of our lower body. If the ankles, knees, and hips bow outward, the entire foot moves into a full arched position. When the ankle, knees, and hips fall inward, the foot subsequently collapses and the arch flattens out.

We can manipulate the position of our feet by setting our hips and knees in a good position prior to initiating our squat. This connected lower-body movement is the physical representation of the joint-by-joint concept we covered in the previous chapter. If one link in the human chain of movement breaks down, the entire structure will be affected.

When we create a good arch in our foot, we inevitably form what we call a tripod foot. The three points of the tripod consists of the heel, the base of the first toe, and the base of the fifth toe. Our foot is basically like a three-wheeled motorcycle. Our goal when squatting should be to maintain the arch of our feet and have our weight distributed evenly—like the three wheels of a motorcycle. If all of the wheels are in contact with the ground, we get more power. If one wheel is off the ground or if the body bottoms out, power is lost and the motorcycle breaks down. When our foot is out of position (arch collapse), stability and power are lost.

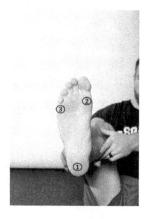

Try this simple test at home. Take your shoes off and assume a squat stance. With our shoes off, we should all have our feet relatively straightforward. Notice what position your feet are in. Do you have equal weight on each of the three contact tripod points? Is your arch in a good position or has it already collapsed? The goal is to become aware of how your foot is functioning.

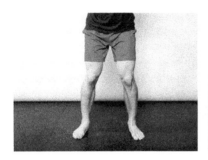 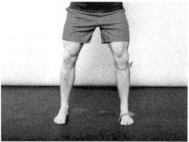

From this position, squeeze your butt muscles and drive your knees out to the side while keeping your big toe in contact with the ground. Notice what position your feet are now in. Did anything change? By setting our knees in a stable position, we naturally bring our feet into a good position.

As you squat, don't just think about keeping your knees in line with your feet. Do your best to maintain your arch and the tripod foot. Keep your foot strong and stable. Don't let the arch collapse. Notice how this feels? Your squat should feel more stable.

If you can pass this test with a bodyweight squat, try it again with a pistol squat. The pistol squat challenges the body to a greater degree than a bodyweight squat. The goal with this activity is to increase our awareness of our feet position during the squat and the pistol squat. Every athlete, regardless of foot type, should be capable of performing a double- and single-leg squat barefoot while maintaining a stable foot. An inability to do so highlights a crack in the movement foundation. Left unchecked, this crack will wreak havoc on athletes' barbell lifts and affect his or her skilled field movements.

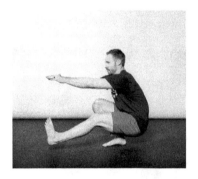

Once we can get our athletes to adopt a better position with their feet, a lot of the other movement problems they have will take care of themselves. The body naturally starts to assume better positions because it is now moving from a stable platform. In doing so, we not only improve movement quality but also decrease pain and improve our performance. This all starts with solidifying our base.

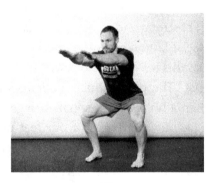

Chapter 5
The Mobile Ankle

5.1 Screening for Ankle Stiffness

In the last chapter, we discussed how creating a "tripod" foot ensures proper stability for our squat from the bottom up. If you recall the joint-by-joint concept, the stable foot sets the foundation for our mobile ankle. This is the topic of the current chapter.

Despite the occasional ankle sprain, our ankle is naturally a fairly stable joint. It is prone to become stiff and immobile. For this reason, the role of the ankle is movement or mobility. When our ankle loses its ability to move, it affects the rest of the body. The foot below becomes unstable, and therefore the natural arch of the foot collapses. The knee above also becomes unstable. When we squat, an unstable knee will often wobble and fall inward. These are only the immediate effects of an immobile ankle. Eventually, a stiff ankle could negatively impact the rest of the body. Entire movement patterns can be thrown out of whack due to stiff ankles.

In order to perform a full-depth squat, our bodies require a certain amount of ankle mobility. Unless you are performing a low-bar back squat, the knee must be able to move forward over your toes. This forward knee movement comes from the ankle, and it is called dorsiflexion. You can measure dorsiflexion by drawing a line with the shin and another line with the outside of the foot. The smaller or more closed the angle is, the more ankle dorsiflexion the athlete has. A restriction in this motion is where most athletes run into trouble.

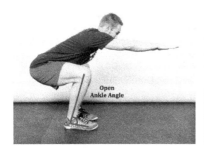
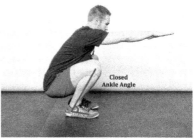

Stiff ankles are often a culprit behind our squat problems. Do your feet point outward when you squat even when you try your hardest to keep the toes forward? Can you remain upright in the bottom of your snatch or clean? Do your knees constantly fall inward when you perform a pistol squat? All of these movement problems can be related to poor ankle mobility.

I want to introduce a simple way to assess our ankles. This screening will tell us if we have full mobility or if our movement problems are a result of a problem somewhere else in the body.

This test is called the half-kneeling dorsiflexion test. This specific test has been used numerous times in research to assess ankle mobility.[1] Physical therapist Dr. Mike Reinold recommended this screening for its ability to provide reliable results without the need for a trained specialist.[2]

Find a wall and kneel close to it with your shoes off. Use a tape measure and place your big toe five inches from the wall. From this position, push your knee forward, attempting to touch the wall with your knee. Your heel must stay in contact with the ground.

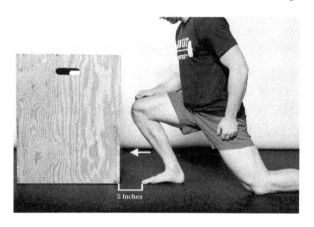

Movement Checklist:

Pass			Fail
	Knee can touch the wall at five-inch or more distance	Knee unable to touch wall at five-inch distance	
	Heels remain firmly planted	Heels pull off from ground	
	Knees aligned with feet	Knees collapse inward (Valgus collapse) in order to touch wall	
	No pain noted	Pain noted	

Did you have checkmarks in the "pass" column? If you could touch your knee to the wall at a distance of five inches while keeping your knee in line with your foot, you show adequate mobility in the ankle.[3]

However, if you had any checks in the "fail" column for this screening, you have a dorsiflexion mobility restriction. This restriction could be either a soft-tissue restriction or a joint-mobility problem—or both.

With the joint-by-joint concept, we can learn to assess the body in a different fashion than we have in the past. Always assess movement first. If you found a problem in your single- or double-leg squat, we can then use different tools (such as the half-kneeling dorsiflexion screening) to find out the cause of the breakdown. By addressing ankle mobility issues, we can improve the overall quality of our movements.

5.2 Joint Restriction or Soft-Tissue Stiffness?

Let's now discuss the results of the ankle mobility screening. After performing the test, what did you notice? Did you pass? Don't worry if you failed. You are a part of a large majority of athletes with stiff ankles. It is important to understand the different reasons for developing stiffness at the ankle so that we can appropriately treat the problem. There is no one-size-fits-all approach to fixing stiff ankles.

Stiff ankles are primarily caused by two different factors.

1. Joint restriction
2. Soft-tissue restrictions

Joint Restriction

Joint restriction is simply defined as a loss of space between the bones that connect at the ankle. Essentially, they stop moving appropriately over one another. Bone spurs or abnormal calcifications within the joint are some of the main reasons for this type of block.[4] They usually develop after trauma, such as a previously sprained ankle. Old age can also contribute to a bony block.

A common result of joint restriction is impingement of the ankle joint. This is usually felt as a "pinching" or "blocked" sensation in the front portion of the ankle during the ankle mobility screen.

In the book *Anatomy for Runners*, physical therapist Jay Dicharry uses a perfect metaphor for describing how these types of restrictions change our movement patterns.[5] If you have ever driven your car through a European-inspired roundabout, you know that you can't just drive straight through the intersection. You have to go around the center island.

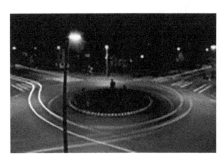
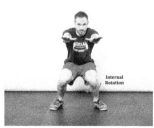

An ankle with full mobility will allow the tibia to move freely on the foot. Think of this like a car being able to move straight through an intersection. A bony block is like a roundabout in the intersection. When the car enters the intersection, it must now go around the island in order to proceed on its previous route. Essentially, our lower leg spins off its normal route and falls inward. As our lower leg goes around the bony block, the knee is pulled inward. Movement breaks down.

If you could not pass the ankle-mobility screen and you felt a "pinch" or "block" in the front of your ankle, there is a possibility that you have a bony block. We can use ankle-mobilization exercises in order to fix this type of stiffness.

Soft-Tissue Restriction
Soft-tissue restrictions at the ankle joint include muscles (gastrocnemius, soleus, tibialis posterior) and fascia. These structures can become stiff and inflexible over time. For example, a sedentary lifestyle or wearing high heels often can cause these muscles to become stiff and tight.

Fascia, a type of connective tissue, weaves its way around our entire body. Fascia is like a spider web that spans from the top of our head to the bottom of our feet. It wraps around and envelops bones, muscles, organs, nerves…basically everything!

When we move often and with good technique, the fascia surrounding muscles stays pliable and elastic. If you viewed fascia under a microscope, it would appear in an organized weave pattern.[6] This weave design allows the soft tissues in our body to glide easily over one another in a smooth fashion.

Inactivity and poor movement disrupts this weave pattern. The once organized pattern ends up looking more like a random scribble drawn by a two-year-old kid with crayons. Not only are the fascial fibers now arranged in a complete mess, but also they actually lose their elasticity and stop gliding easily over one another.[7] When this happens, natural flexibility is restricted and movement is limited.

Earlier I mentioned an analogy about a bony block as equivalent to a roundabout; well, a soft-tissue restriction is more like a traffic jam. As your knee tries to move forward over the toe, it runs into a congested mess and is basically halted in its track. When this happens, our body will do one of two things.

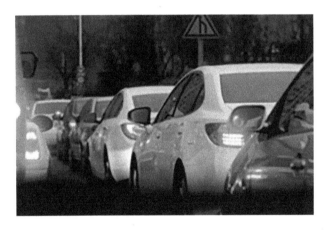

First, the knee will stop moving forward and somewhere else in the body will have to move. This is what happens when we see a lifter's chest collapse to get deeper in his or her squat. The other option is even worse. The knee will take a path of least resistance and fall inward. This is basically like a car going off-roading to get around the traffic jam. When the ankle rolls in, it takes the knee with it. Again, movement breaks down.

These types of limitations will usually be felt as tightness in the calf or heel cord during the ankle-mobility screen. If this is the case for you, we will go about addressing this restriction later with two different tools: stretching and foam rolling.

5.3 Mobility Corner

There are many great ideas available today to improve ankle mobility. In this section of the chapter, I want to share with you some of my favorites as a part of my three-step process in dealing with ankle stiffness.

1. Mobilize
2. Foam roll
3. Stretch

Ankle Mobilizations

A restriction in joint mobility should be the first area to address. During the ankle-mobility screen, a "pinch" or "block" sensation felt in the front of your ankle usually signifies this type of restriction. These types of restrictions will not resolve themselves on their own with conventional stretching and foam rolling. Therefore, if you had a pinching sensation during the ankle-mobility screening, it needs to be addressed first before moving on to possible soft-tissue stiffness.

One of the easiest ways to create mobility in restricted joints on your own is to use a band mobilization. The rubber material of the band is elastic and strong enough to affect the tough joint capsules.

Band distraction joint mobilizations simply help increase the way our bones glide over each other. A joint glide is sustained while the athlete actively moves into the specific range of motion we are trying to change. If we look at the ankle, the talus bone of the foot moves backward as the shin moves forward into dorsiflexion as we squat. In order to help improve this movement to increase mobility, the band must help push the talus bone backward.[7, 8] Often, athletes will have the band placed too high on the ankle. This backward pull on the tibia will actually do the opposite of what we want to achieve.

These types of mobilizations (simply termed *mobilizations with movement*) have been used for years by physical therapists. The goal is to alleviate any once-painful or pinching feelings deep in the joint.

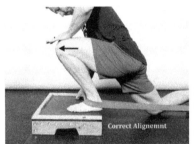
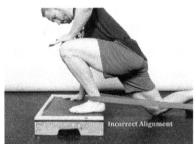

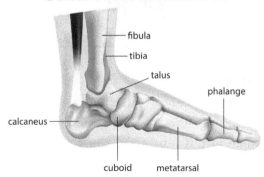

Bones of the Human Foot

Foam Rolling

Once joint restrictions have been addressed, the next step is to clear up any soft-tissue stiffness. This starts with using a foam roller. I usually recommended athletes spend at least two minutes on each area they are trying to address with a foam roller. Every athlete should spend time each day using this tool.

Start by moving slowly up and down the lower leg muscles until you find a tender area. Pause on this area and "tack it down" with your opposite leg for about ten seconds before moving to find another spot. You can also add in some ankle pumps during this pause to increase the effectiveness.

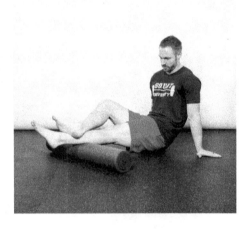

Soft-Tissue Stretching

Once foam rolling is complete, stretching the muscles is the next step to addressing soft-tissue restrictions. The classic ankle stretch is a good go-to in order to make some quick improvements. Before starting your workout, using this stretch after foam rolling is a great way to decrease any amount of stiffness in the lower leg.

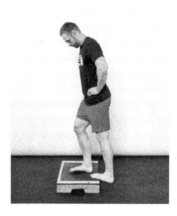

Another version of this stretch is one I like to use prior to training sessions that include any form of barbell squatting. It is very position specific and therefore has good carry-over to the exact movements we are going to perform. To start, drop into a deep goblet squat. This can be performed with either a kettle bell or a weighted plate. From this position, shift your weight onto one foot. Push your knee far forward over your toe until you feel a stretch in the lower calf. After holding for about ten seconds, shift to the other leg.

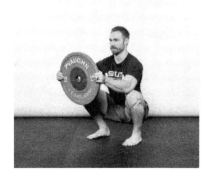
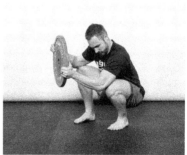

Test-Retest

After you have addressed your stiff ankles, it's time to check on the progress you have made. Always employ a test-retest strategy when performing mobility exercises. This allows you to see if the tools you are using are effective in addressing the change you desire.

Performing the ankle mobility screening is a great way to measure and see if you have made any change. However, in the end our goal is to make a lasting change in our overall movement pattern of the squat. For this reason, it is just as important to see how any improvements in ankle mobility have affected your squat. After working on your ankle mobility, perform a deep squat. Then, perform a deep single-leg pistol squat. Do you notice anything different?

While not everyone has the same reasons for ankle stiffness, using these tools can be the first step in helping make a lasting change and improving your squat and pistol squat technique.

Notes

1. K. Bennell, R. Talbot, H. Wajswelner, W. Techovanich, and D. Kelly, "Intra-rater and Inter-rater Reliability of a Weight-bearing Lunge Measure of Ankle Dorsiflexion," *Australian Journal of Physiotherapy* 44, no. 3 (1998): 175–80.
2. M. Reinold, "Ankle Mobility Exercises to Improve Dorsiflexion," accessed on December 1, 2015, MikeReinold.com.
3. G. W. Hess, "Ankle Impingement Syndromes: A Review of Etiology and Related Implications," *Foot Ankle Specialist* 4, no. 5 (2011): 290–97.
4. J. Dicharry, *Anatomy for Runners* (New York: Skyhorse Publishing, 2012).
5. R. Schleip and D. G. Muller, "Training Principles for Fascial Connective Tissues: Scientific Foundation and Suggested Practical Applications," *Journal of Bodywork & Movement Therapies* 17 (2013): 103–15.
6. T. A. Jarvinen, L. Jozsa, P. Kannus, T. L. Jarvinen, and M. Jarvinen, "Organization and Distribution of Intramuscular Connective Tissue in Normal and Immobilized Skeletal Muscles: An Immunohisto Chemical, Polarization and Scanning Electron Microscopic Study," *Journal of Muscle Research and Cell Motility* 23, no. 3 (2002): 245–54.
7. B. Vicenzino, M. Branjerdporn, P. Teys, and K. Jordan, "Initial Changes in Posterior Talar Glide and Dorsiflexion of the Ankle after Mobilization with Movement in Individuals with Recurrent Ankle Sprain," *Manual Therapy* 9, no. 2 (May 2004): 77–82.

8. A. Reid, T. B. Birmingham, and G. Alcock, "Efficacy of Mobilization with Movement for Patients with Limited Dorsiflexion after Ankle Sprain: A Crossover Trial," *Physiotherapy Canada* 59, no. 3 (2007): 166–72.

Photo Attribution
1. Bones of Human Foot: BlueRIngMedia/Shutterstock.com

Chapter 6
The Stable Knee

The knee is basically a hinge that is stuck between the ankle and hip joints. In order to reach full depth, we require the knee to fully hinge open and close. This motion is described as flexion and extension. It can be measured by drawing a line on the outside of the thigh and the lower leg. The smaller or more closed the angle is, the more flexion the knee has.

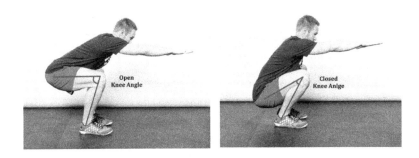

Most athletes do not have an issue in achieving full knee flexion. The main problem we see is the inability to control the knee during dynamic movements like the squat. When I say unstable, what I mean is that often athletes have a difficult time keeping their knee in a steady and unwavering position. Athletes who develop pain in their knees or sustain traumatic injuries (such as the torn ACL) tend to have unstable knees. When we view the squat from the front, we see the knee tends to wobble around like crazy and at times rotate inward, collapsing toward the midline of the body.

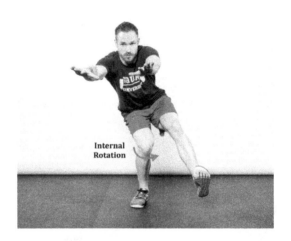

The ideal position of our knees is to be in direct alignment with the feet. An effective cue is "drive the knees wide." With this cue, an athlete can establish the knee-over-toes alignment during the squat. The knee is considered to be unstable anytime its position deviates from this ideal alignment. The inward cave-in of the knee (labeled a valgus collapse) is the most common fault we see. If the foot is placed in the stable tripod position during the entire lift, there is no way for the knee to collapse in or out.

The knee joint would therefore benefit from increased stability to limit this inward collapse. Improving the control of our knees allows us to avoid injury while increasing the efficiency of our movement. By increasing efficiency of our movements, we can produce more power and increase strength. Who wouldn't want more power and more strength and to avoid injuries?

6.1 Screening for Knee Instability

Let's talk about screening the knee. Before we enter this discussion, there is one point I would like to make. If an athlete presents with stiff ankles and/or hips, this issue will likely result in an unstable knee. For this reason, always address the hip and ankle prior to screening the knee. If you skip the hip and ankle, any knee stability we try to establish will be short lived.

After clearing the ankle and hips, we can now focus on the stability of the knee. We need to view our squat in both double- and single-leg stance. The double-leg squat can sometimes mask any stability issues. Therefore, I would like to look at pistol squats on one leg. Often times, an athlete may be proficient in a double-leg squat but then demonstrate valgus collapse with the pistol squat.

To start our assessment, stand with your feet at a comfortable width with your toes in a relatively straightforward position. Perform a deep squat. Next, assume a single-leg stance and perform a deep pistol squat. What do you notice? Does your knee wobble around and fall inward or can you keep it in line with your feet?

It can be helpful to also test the loaded squat. The weighted barbell allows us to test the competency of our movement. The more weight on the bar, the higher the demand on the body.

Very often I see athletes who can perform the perfect bodyweight squat but when they perform a weighted back squat, their form turns to crap. It is never okay or justifiable to lose good technique to achieve a new one-rep-max personal record.

The weight on the bar means nothing if our technique goes to crap! If the knees collapse during a maximum squat attempt, the risk of injury greatly increases. Period.

In the past year, there have been a number of world records set in the sport of weightlifting. Tremendous weight moved in the blink of an eye. All of them were performed with good technique. These weightlifters spend day after day perfecting their movement with the barbell. No matter if you're performing a world-record snatch or a simple bodyweight squat, good technique is a necessity. If you want to stay healthy and reach your true strength potential, focusing on stabilizing the knees is vital.

6.2 Corrective Exercise Corner

I now want to introduce to you my three-step process for improving knee stability.

1. Correct technique
2. Touchdown progression
3. Strengthen the hips

<u>*Correct Technique*</u>
Our first move in addressing unstable knees is working on correct technique. Some athletes have never been shown how to

squat correctly. At times, correcting squat technique is all they need to stabilize the knees.

One of the most common cues that I like to use is "drive the knees out." This prompt teaches athletes to engage their hips properly and keep the knees from collapsing inward as they squat. However, it must be followed with "keep your feet firmly planted."

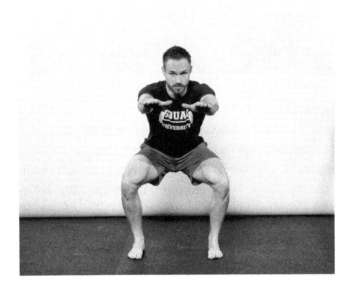

Pushing the knees out too far without maintaining the tripod foot can be an issue as well. Their weight will shift to the outside of their foot, allowing the base of the big toe to become unglued to the floor. As long as the foot remains firmly planted on the ground in the tripod position, the "knees out" cue is a great starting point.

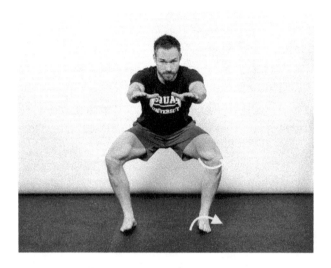

The second cue I will use to help stabilize the knee is "drive the hips back." One of the absolutes of squatting is proper engagement of our posterior chain (primarily our glute max) prior to starting the descent. This occurs by driving the hips backward in a motion called the hip hinge. You need more hip hinge with the low-bar squat when compared to the overhead squat or the front squat.

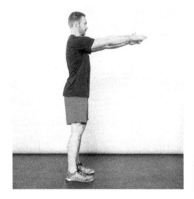
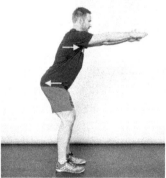

Whether you're performing a low-bar back squat or overhead squat, you must engage the posterior chain prior to starting the squat. Loading our hips (the powerhouse of our body) will take pressure off the knees. Not engaging the posterior chain will increase the likelihood of the knees wobbling around.

Touchdown Progression

If the athlete is unable to correct knee instability with cueing, it's time to take a different approach. This means moving onto one leg and perfecting the pistol squat. You would be surprised by how many powerful athletes are capable of squatting a tremendous amount of weight but unable to perform a simple single-leg squat.

In the strength game, we often forget about training on a single leg because we spend so much time working on improving our numbers on the main core lifts: the squat, deadlift, clean, and snatch. In doing so, it is easy to unknowingly develop weakness in some areas of our body. Challenging yourself with single-leg squats can illuminate any deficits you have. Not only that, but performing single-leg activities will work on balance. Every athlete needs to work on balance.

By starting small and progressing appropriately, we can see a dramatic change in the ability to control the knee. In order to do this, we will use a small box or a weight plate. Starting with a lower surface, we can then work our way up to a full pistol squat.

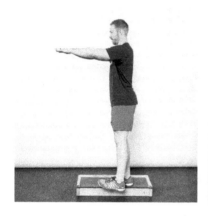 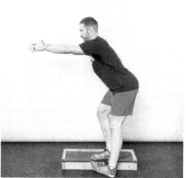

Start by using a four-inch box. If you're at the gym, you can stack two weighted plates on top of each other. Assume a single-leg stance on top of the box or plates. From this position, drive your hips backward and bring your chest forward. This movement allows you to engage your posterior chain. If you do this correctly, you should feel slight tension in your glute and hamstring muscles. Bringing your chest forward while driving the hips back will bring you into a balanced position with your bodyweight over the middle of your foot.

Keeping the knee in line with your foot, squat down until your opposite heel gently taps the floor before returning to the starting position. If you are doing this exercise correctly, you will feel your butt muscles working hard after a few reps. You should not feel any pain or stiffness in your knees.

When you're performing this exercise, try to keep your shin as vertical as possible. Allowing the knees to slide forward too soon will increase the pressure on the joint and the susceptibility of caving in. Eventually, the knee will have to move forward as the depth of the single-leg squat increases. However, there should be little forward movement of the knee during this initial small box.

As the four-inch box becomes easier and easier, increase the difficulty by moving to a higher box or adding more weights. A higher box will demand more control from the knee. Eventually, the goal will be to perform a full pistol squat with a good technique.

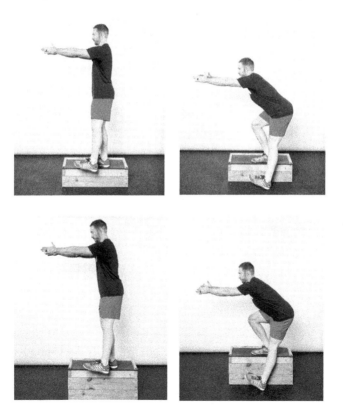

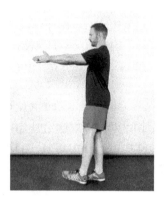 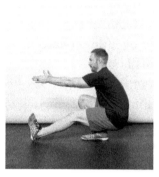

Strengthen the Hips

The lateral hip muscles (primarily the gluteus medius) play an important role in stabilizing our knee. When we squat or we land from a jump or run, these muscles ensure the knees stay in line with the foot and don't cave in. Strengthening these muscles can improve the ability to stabilize the knee.

My favorite exercise to strengthen the hips is called the lateral band walk. This exercise is performed exactly how it sounds. To start, place an elastic band around your ankles. I'm a fan of the exercise bands from Perform Better. If you can't find one, a longer monster band can be used (tension will just be applied through the hold).

The starting position is the same three-step process we go through every time we squat. Place the feet in a comfortable position with the toes relatively straightforward. Next, ensure the feet are in a stable tripod position. Drive the knees out to the side to bring them into alignment with the feet. Lastly, engage the posterior chain by driving the hips slightly backward and bringing the chest forward to remain in balance.

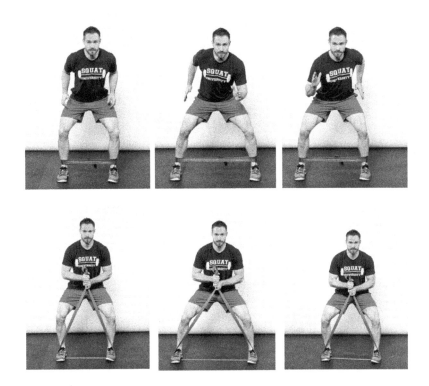

From this position, start walking sideways with small steps. Make sure constant tension is applied the entire time from the band. After walking fifteen to twenty feet, stop and come back the other way. Eventually, you should start to feel fatigue in your lateral hip muscles.

Test-Retest

Improvements in knee stability are not always easily attained. Instability is something that has been learned and programmed into the body for some time. The longer you have moved poorly, the longer it will take to learn how to move correctly.

Chapter 7
The Mobile Hip

The hip is another area of the body that tends to develop stiffness. A sedentary lifestyle and excessive sitting are a couple reasons why we develop stiff hips. Limited range of motion at the hips can limit our ability to squat to full depth. Most of us could benefit from working on our hip mobility issues.

When the hips lack adequate mobility, a few things can happen. First, the knees will lose stability and start to bow inward. Second, the lower back will fail to remain stable and collapse into a rounded position. Each of these movement problems wreaks havoc on our power and increases our risk for injury.

Adequate hip flexion is needed to reach a full-depth squat (hips below parallel). You can measure flexion of the hip by drawing a line with the torso and another line with the outside of the upper leg. The smaller or more closed the angle is, the more hip flexion the athlete has.

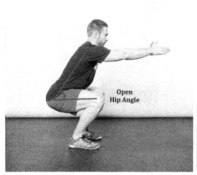 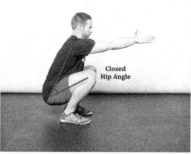

7.1 Screening for Hip Stiffness

If you are unable to squat to full depth with toes relatively straightforward, hip mobility is likely a limiting factor. I now want to introduce one of my favorite tools for assessing hip mobility. It is called the Thomas test.[1]

This test is performed while lying on your back. The Thomas test's main purpose is to look for tightness of iliopsoas (hip flexor muscle), rectus femoris (quad muscle), or iliotibial band. All of these soft-tissue structures can contribute to hip mobility issues.

Start by standing next to a bed or a bench. Your hips should be in contact with the edge. Grab one of your knees and pull it toward your chest as you gently fall backward. The knee you grab should be pulled as close to your chest as possible. As you lie on your back while holding onto your knee, allow your other leg to relax completely.

What position does your body end up in? Having a friend help you with this screening is extremely beneficial. Once you screen one leg, perform the same movement on the opposite leg and see what you find.

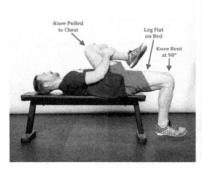
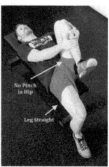

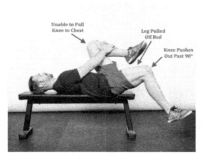
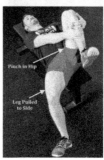

Movement Checklist:

Pass			Fail
	Able to pull knee fully to chest	Unable to pull knee to chest	
	Able to keep opposite leg flat on bed	Unable to keep opposite leg flat on bed	
	Opposite leg lies in a straight position on bed	Opposite leg is turned out to the side of body	
	Opposite knee is flexed and relaxed	Opposite knee is relatively straight and tight	

Did you have checks in every box of the "pass" column? If so, you show adequate hip flexion mobility. However, if you had any checks in the "fail" column for this screening, you have a hip mobility restriction.

If you were unable to pull your knee fully to your chest, we are dealing with a possible hip flexion mobility issue. This could be caused by a number of factors including tight or restricted soft tissues or even hip capsule restrictions.

If you were unable to pull one of your legs as far toward your chest as the other, you have a possible asymmetry in hip mobility. This is a red flag. Asymmetries are very important to take care of as they can negatively influence barbell squats. Often these small side-to-side differences go undiagnosed. Left untreated, asymmetries can lead to overuse injuries.

The Thomas test also allows us to screen for mobility restrictions in the opposite hip. An inability to keep your opposite leg flat on the bed and in a straight line can also point toward hip stiffness.

Remember to always assess movement first. If you found a problem in your single- or double-leg squat, we can then use different tools (such as the Thomas test) to find out the cause of the breakdown in the movement.

7.2 Joint Restriction or Soft-Tissue Stiffness?

With adequate mobility at the hips, our knees and lower back remain stable. The main idea behind the joint-by-joint concept is that our bodies consist of ever-connecting parts. A weak link in our chain of movement will cause a breakdown in the entire system. Stiff hips limit our ability to squat with good technique.

Let's now discuss the results of the Thomas test. After performing the test, what did you notice? Did you pass? Don't worry if you failed! It is important to understand the different reasons for developing stiffness at the hips so that we can appropriately treat the problem. There is no one-size-fits-all approach to fixing stiff hips.

Stiff hips are primarily caused by two different factors.

1. Joint restriction
2. Soft-tissue restrictions

Joint Restriction

Joint restriction is simply defined as a loss of space between the bones that connect at the hip. Essentially, they stop moving appropriately over one another. This tightness creates a roadblock in the joint. This bony blockade halts the forward movement of the femur (thigh bone) in the hip joint when we try to bring our knee to our chest (like in the Thomas test). This movement restriction is called FAI or femoroacetabular impingement.[2] This mobility problem is usually the result of repetitive strain, such as the wear and tear effects of pushing through pinching pain in the bottom of a squat. It can also be caused by long-term adaptation to a sedentary lifestyle.

If you had difficulty pulling your knee up to your chest and felt a "pinch" in the hip, there is a possibility that you have FAI. We previously discussed the analogy about the roundabout in a restricted ankle joint. With FAI, the femur will actually hit a "blockade," causing that pinching sensation in the front of the hip.

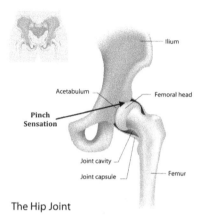

The Hip Joint

Our bodies, however, are a little smarter than we think and will naturally compensate our movement pattern in order to get the job done. Because of the hip restriction, the lower back is forced to move! This lower back movement decreases our stability during squats, preventing optimal power and strength gains.

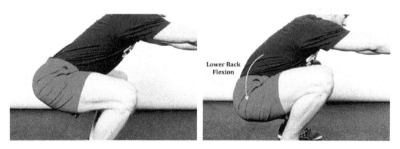

We can go about resolving this problem through two methods. First, we can use joint mobilization exercises to increase space in the hip joint. Second, we will ensure our posterior chain (glute and hamstring muscles) is working efficiently. An inability to properly activate the glutes during movements like the squat is commonly seen.

Soft-Tissue Restriction

Soft-tissue restrictions at the hip joint include muscles (iliopsoas and quadriceps), the IT band, and fascia. These structures can become stiff and inflexible over time. For example, a sedentary lifestyle such as sitting for long periods will often lead to stiffness and tightness. Excessive inactivity can cause fascia to lose its elasticity, thereby making it difficult for surrounding tissues to glide easily over one another. Plain and simple, excessive sitting decreases our natural hip flexibility and degrades normal movement patterns (such as the squat).

This type of limitation will usually be felt as tightness in the front or lateral part of the free hip during the Thomas test. Some common findings during the Thomas test are that the free leg remains off the bed and falls out to the side or your knee is unable to relax into a bent position. If this is the case for you, we will go about addressing these types of restrictions with two different tools: stretching and foam rolling.

Hip mobility is a very important aspect in achieving a full-depth squat. Stiff hips decrease our ability to properly activate the appropriate muscles in our hips. Essentially, we bleed out a good amount of power during heavy squats. Understanding the cause of our restricted hip mobility is the first step in establishing effective ways to fix the problem.

7.3 Mobility Corner

I now want to share with you my four-step process in dealing with hip stiffness.

1. Mobilize
2. Foam roll
3. Stretch
4. Posterior-chain activation

Hip Mobilizations

A restriction in joint mobility should be the first area to address. During the Thomas test, a "pinching" sensation felt in the front of the hip when pulling your knee to your chest indicates possible impingement. This sensation is felt when the femur hits the joint "blockade," halting the movement at the hip joint. These types of restrictions will not resolve with conventional stretching and foam rolling. Therefore, any pinching sensation in the hip joint must be addressed first before moving onto possible soft-tissue stiffness.

One of the easiest ways to improve joint restrictions on your own is to use a band for mobilization. The rubber material of the band is elastic and strong enough to affect the tough joint capsule of the hip.

Band distraction joint mobilizations assist with the way our bones glide over each other. A joint glide is sustained while the athlete actively moves into the specific range of motion we are trying to improve. During the squat, the end of our femur glides backward in our hip joint as our thigh moves toward our chest. These types of mobilizations (simply termed *mobilizations with movement*) have been used for years by physical therapists. The goal is to alleviate any painful or pinching feelings deep in the joint.

Start with the band pulled close to your hip joint. Assume a lunge position with the band around your forward leg. The band should be pulling laterally in this position. Research describes the lateral banded mobilization as the most effective way to alleviate a pinching sensation in the front of your hip during a deep squat.[3]

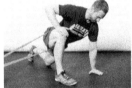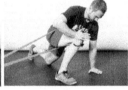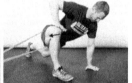

From this position, rock your knee inward and back ten times. With enough tension on the band, this should cause a light stretching sensation in your lateral hip. You are performing a small lateral glide of your femur in the hip socket. This is providing more space for the femur in the socket and eliminating the amount of bone-on-bone contact that creates the pinching sensation in the bottom of the squat. Next, push your knee out to the side and back. In these positions, squeeze your glute muscles for a few seconds and then relax.

Foam Rolling
Once joint restrictions have been addressed, the next step is to clear up any soft-tissue stiffness. This starts with using a foam roller. I usually recommend athletes spend at least two minutes

on each area they are trying to address. Every athlete should foam roll on a daily basis!

Our goal with the foam roller is to decrease the stiffness the Thomas test was able to expose. This means addressing our hip flexors, quads, and lateral hips. Start by moving slowly up and down the lower leg muscles until you find a tender area. Pause on this area and "tack it down" with your bodyweight for about ten seconds before moving again.

I like to use the analogy of kneading bread with a rolling pin. You want to use the foam roller to knead your tissues, rolling back and forth in small, rhythmical movements. Lying on the roller and moving quickly in large passes will have little effect on your stiff tissues. You can also add in active knee movement during this pause to increase the effectiveness.

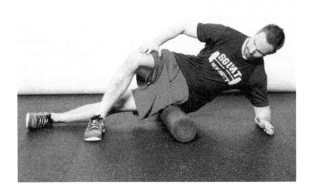

Soft-Tissue Stretching
Once foam rolling is complete, stretching the muscles is the

next step. My first go-to stretch for opening up our hips and improving our mobility prior to squatting is called the "world's greatest stretch."

This stretch has four parts to it. First, start by assuming a deep lunge position with your left leg forward. Squeeze your glutes and drive your hips toward the floor. This movement should cause a stretch to be felt in the front of the right hip. Second, drop your left elbow to the ground. Hold for five seconds.

Next, use your elbow or hand to drive your left knee out to the side. Make sure to keep your foot firmly planted on the ground. Finally, rotate the entire upper body up and to the left, ending with the left arm in the air. This last movement helps address the mobility of the thoracic (midspine) that is also prone to stiffness.

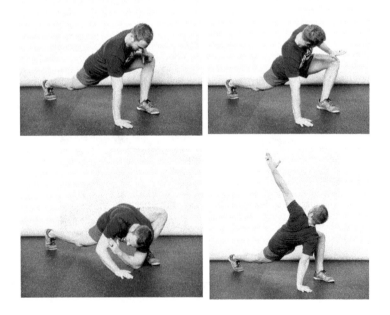

Another stretch I like to use is the half-kneeling hip flexor stretch. This is a great tool for addressing the muscles in the front of our hip. The hip flexors and/or quads can become excessively tight as an adaptation to sitting all day.

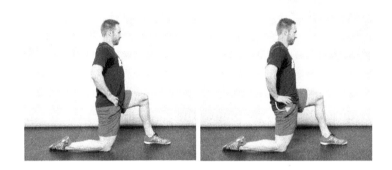

To start this movement, assume a kneeling position. While keeping your chest upright, squeeze your glutes and pull your pelvis under your body. This should elicit a good stretch in the front of your hip. Hold this stretch for ten seconds before relaxing.

The last stretch I want to share with you is a more position-specific movement and therefore has good carryover to the squat itself. To start, drop into a deep goblet squat. This can be performed with either a kettle bell or a weighted plate. Holding a weight in front of us allows us to worry less about balance and more on the deep-squat position we want to improve.

After reaching full depth, drive your knees out to the side of your feet as far as possible with your elbows. Make sure the entire time that your feet stay firmly planted on the floor in the good tripod position. Driving the knees out to the side with your elbows will increase the stretch felt in your hips.

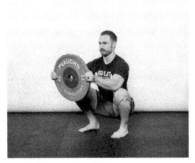 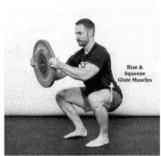

As you open your hips up in this position, you can also work on activating your glutes. The glutes are the primary muscle group that drives us up and out of the bottom of the squat. While you sit in the bottom of the goblet squat, try to squeeze your glutes and drive your knees out to the side as hard as you can for a few seconds (make sure to keep your feet flat). Next, relax and allow your body to drop into the stretch again.

This specific type of stretch is called a "contract-relax" technique. Physical therapists and strength coaches commonly use these techniques because they are so effective in improving our mobility compared to the classic long-duration stretches. After holding for about thirty seconds to a minute, stand up and take a break. I like to perform this movement two or three times before moving on.

Posterior-Chain Activation
The inability to properly activate the posterior chain (glutes and hamstrings) during the squat is a common finding in athletes. For this reason, I recommend athletes perform a quick exercise to prime these muscles after addressing their mobility issues.

The movement I want to show you is called unilateral abduction.

The layperson's term for this exercise is *banded lateral kicks*. To start, place an elastic band around your ankles. Next, assume an athletic single-leg stance. Once in this position, push the hips backward and allow the chest to move forward. This small movement allows us to engage our posterior chain and remain balanced. The cue I like to use for every squat (even small ones like this) to solidify this idea is "squat with the hips—not with the knees."

Once we are in position, kick the nonstance leg out to the side and back in a slow and controlled manner. The distance the leg moves out to the side is not our main concern. Focus on keeping the stance leg in a stable and unwavering position during the entire exercise. This exercise not only primes the glutes for the squatting we will perform after, but it will help address core and knee stability problems. Perform two to three sets of fifteen repetitions. This should leave your lateral hips fatigued!

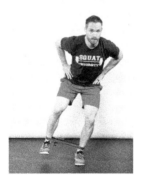 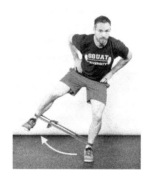

Test-Retest
After you have addressed your stiff hips, it's time to check and see the progress you have made. Always employ a test-retest

strategy when performing mobility exercises. This allows you to see if the tools you are using are effective in addressing the change you desire.

Performing a deep bodyweight squat is a great way to assess any changes. Also attempt a deep pistol squat. Do you notice anything different? Our goal is to make a lasting change in our overall movement pattern of the squat. Mobility tools are only effective if they carry over to an exercise we're trying to work on.

My hope for this chapter is to give you the tools necessary to address any hip-stiffness problems. If you want to remain competitive or move around pain free, it is vital that you improve and maintain good hip mobility.

Notes

1. D. Harvey, "Assessment of the Flexibility of Elite Athletes Using the Modified Thomas Test," *British Journal of Sports Medicine* 32, no. 1 (1998): 68–70.
2. M. Leunig, P. E. Beaule, and R Ganz, "The Concept of Femoroacetabular Impingement: Current Status and Future Perspectives," *Clinical Orthopedics and Related Research* 467, no. 3 (March 2009): 616–22.
3. M. P. Reiman and J. W. Matheson, "Restricted Hip Mobility: Clinical Suggestion for Self-mobilization and Muscle Re-education," *International Journal of Sports Physical Therapy* 8, no. 5 (October 2013): 729–40.

Photo Attribution

1. The Hip Joint: AlilaMedicalMedia/Shutterstock.com

Chapter 8
The Stable Core

All too often, I see athletes who go about training their core in the wrong way. Many coaches are still under the impression that by strengthening the muscles of the core, stability will be enhanced. For this reason, it is common to see athletes still performing endless crunches or hypers off a glute-ham machine. While these muscles do need to be strong, isolation strengthening in this manner actually does little to promote stability that will carry over to helping us squat with better technique.

Core stability is all about timing and coordination. The muscles of our abdomen, back, and hips must work together in order to maintain our lumbar spine in a neutral position as we move. When we combine the action of bracing our core with the power of our breath, we open up the potential to lift tremendous weight.

Corrective exercises for the lower back need to focus on how well we can maintain our back in a stable position and not the number of sit-ups we can perform. Most of us have been training our core the wrong way our entire life!

Before working on core stability, we have to address any hip restrictions we have. Any core stability that we work on will be short lived if we don't have adequate hip mobility.

8.1 Level 1 (Cognitive Stability)

Each level of corrective core-stability exercises is based on the teachings and research from renowned experts Peter O'Sullivan and Dr. Stuart McGill.[1,2] The first stage of training is called the cognitive phase. It focuses on improving our sensation and perception of stability. We need to be able to feel the muscles that should be activated as we brace our core.

Bracing involves activation of all the abdominal muscles of our core (abs, back, diaphragm, and pelvis) to create 360 degrees of stiffness around our spine.[3,4] If bracing is coupled with proper breathing mechanics during heavy squat attempts, stability is enhanced to an even greater degree.[5]

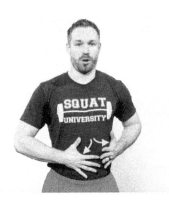

In the past, many experts claimed we needed to only activate the transverse abdominis (a small, flat muscle that runs across the front of our core). However, we have come to realize that activating the transverse abdominis solely is a misdirected attempt to create core stability. This muscle is only one member of the "abdominal team." It is no more important than any of the others that encompass and surround the torso. They must all be equally activated in order to fully support the lower back.

The first exercise I want to introduce is an easy way to learn the bracing process. Focus on feeling the muscles around your entire core activating as we go through this step-by-step process.

Step 1: Lie on the ground with your back to the floor. Your knees can stay bent for comfort.

Step 2: Activate the muscles on all sides of your core, a process called co-contraction. A verbal cue I like to use is to brace yourself as if you were about to receive a punch to the gut. This should create a feeling of firmness around your entire lower torso. Place your hands on your stomach and on your side. You should feel the muscles under your hands tense as they activate. Improper bracing will only activate our rectus abdominus (our six-pack muscle).

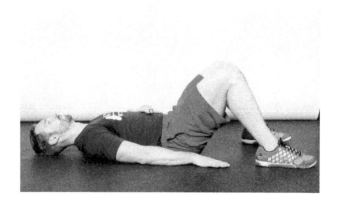

Step 3: Once this pattern has been isolated, we need to train these muscles to work together for an extended period of time (ten to twenty seconds). Stability of our lower back is needed throughout our entire day, not only the few heavy lifts we do in training! Being able to hold this bracing action for a sustained time allows us to increase our stability for increased endurance.

Recommended sets/reps: three sets of ten repetitions.

8.2 Level 2 (Movement Stability)

After learning how to actively co-contract the different muscles of the core, it is time to learn how to maintain that stability as we move. The exercise I want to introduce for this section is the bird-dog progression. During this exercise, focus on how well you are bracing your core. Our ability to maintain stability often falters as soon as movement of the arms or legs is initiated.

Step 1: From the all-fours position (quadruped), place a PVC pipe or cane along the back as shown. At all times, the PVC should be in contact with the back to ensure proper spinal alignment.

Step 2: Once you find the neutral position, re-create that co-contraction of the core you learned from level one. This bracing effort will create the stability needed for the next few steps.

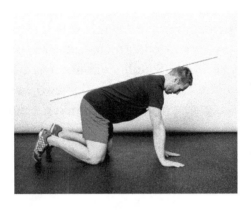

Step 3: Next, lift your arms up toward your head (one at a time) and back toward the starting position by your side. During this arm movement, your lower back should remain in a stable, braced position. It is important to breathe first and then brace your core. Don't hold your breath during this movement. Let your breath out slowly through pursed lips (as if you have a straw in your mouth).

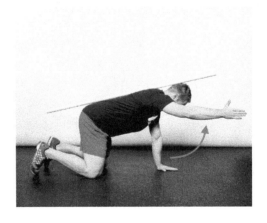

Step 4: Once this stage is mastered, the second step is to perform the movement with one leg at a time. Extend one leg backward as far as possible. Again, this movement should not change the position of your back at all! You should remain solid at all times. If an athlete moves poorly during this stage, his or her lower back will over extend, and he or she will lose contact with the PVC pipe.

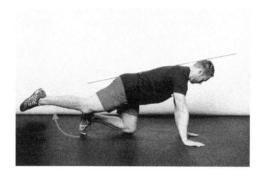

Step 5: The next stage is one where both the legs and arms are moving. Start by moving your right arm and left leg at the same time. This is the standard bird-dog exercise that most people are familiar with.

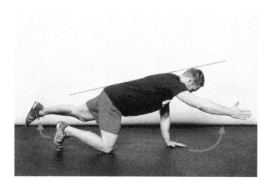

Step 6: The last stage is where the arm and leg on the same side are moving. This stage is very difficult for most people.

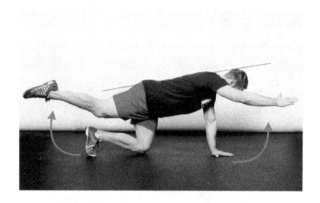

Recommended sets/reps: two sets of ten repetitions at highest level possible without compensation.

8.3 Level 3 (Functional Stability)

Once we develop good awareness of core control/stability, we need to translate it to functional movements. In order to fully grasp true core stability, exercises must eventually be performed in movements that relate to a given sport. One functional core stability exercise I like to use is the "no hands" or "zombie" front squat.

Step 1: Assume a front squat position with the bar held on top of the chest and shoulders.

Step 2: Take your hands away from the bar and hold them out in front of you. This should look like the starting position of the bodyweight squat.

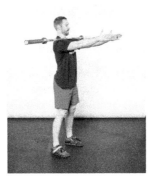

Step 3: Use the proper breathing and bracing pattern to stabilize your core properly. Take a big breath into your stomach followed by a strong brace of your core muscles.

Step 4: Next, perform the front squat to full depth while trying to maintain the bar in the same position. In order to stay balanced, the bar must track over the middle of your foot the entire time. Inability to adequately maintain core stability and stay balanced will force the arms to fall forward. This will cause the bar to roll off the shoulders and drop to the ground.

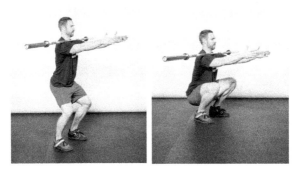

While this corrective exercise can be loaded to increase the difficulty of the movement, the amount of weight added to the bar must be within reasonable amounts. Start with an empty barbell. Once you can do this with ease, progressively add weights to increase the difficulty. Prioritize technique over weight on the bar.

Recommended sets/reps: two to three sets of five repetitions.

Take Away

Proper mechanics during the squat is all about maintaining proper core stability. If core stability is compromised, strength and power are lost.

Notes

1. P. B. O'Sullivan, "Lumbar Segmental 'Instability': Clinical Presentation and Specific Stabilizing Exercise Management," *Manual Therapy* 5, no. 1 (2000): 2–12.
2. S. G. Grenier and S. M. McGill, "Quantification of Lumbar Stability by Using 2 Different Abdominal Activation Strategies," *Archives of Physical Medicine and Rehabilitation* 88, no. 1 (2007): 54–62.
3. M. G. Gardner-Morse and I. A. F. Stokes, "The Effects of Abdominal Muscle Co-activation on Lumbar Spine Stability," *The Spine Journal* 23, no. 1 (1998): 86–92.
4. J. Cholewicki, K. Juluru, and S. M. McGill, "Intra-abdominal Pressure Mechanism for Stabilizing the Lumbar Spine," *Journal of Biomechanics* 32, no. 1 (1999): 13–17.
5. J. M. Willardson, "Core Stability Training: Applications to Sports Conditioning Programs," *Journal of Strength and Conditioning Research* 21, no. 3 (2007): 979–98.

Chapter 9
Overhead Mobility

If I had to single out one exercise that most athletes struggle with, it would be the overhead squat. There are so many variables that could hurt your overhead squat technique.

Mobility/flexibility issues at the thoracic spine, shoulder joint, or chest/back can severely limit an athlete's ability to achieve an overhead squat.

The goal of this chapter is to explain two simple screens you can perform at home to illuminate possible overhead mobility issues.

9.1 Screening Overhead Mobility

The latissimus dorsi or "lats" is one of the largest muscles in the body. It runs from the lower back all the way to your arms. Athletes (especially bodybuilders) with well-defined lats will often have the classic V shape.

When athletes have stiffness in this muscle, it can limit how far they can raise their arm overhead. In his book *Movement*, physical therapist Gray Cook demonstrated the "supine lat stretch" as a simple way to assess flexibility in this muscle.[1]

The Supine Lat Stretch
To start, lie on your back with your arms held above your head.

The palms of your hands should be facing the ceiling. Bring your knees toward your chest as far as possible. Your lower back should be completely flat on the ground. From this position, see if you can move your arms (elbows straight) all the way to the floor above your head.

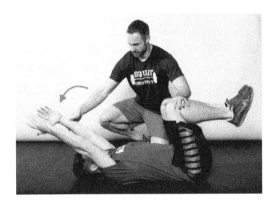

If you were able to lay your arms completely flat on the floor, you more than likely do not have a lat restriction. If your arms dangled above the floor, the next step is straightening your legs out. Make sure to keep your lower back flat on the floor when you do this. Look to see if you can now move your arms closer to the floor above your head.

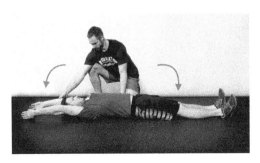

What did you find? If you were able to rest your arms on the floor above your head with your legs now extended, it means you have a possible lat flexibility restriction. By straightening out your legs, the lat muscle is slackened, which should allow your arms to travel down closer to the floor.

If you had only a slight improvement in arm movement and were still unable to rest your arms on the ground with your legs extended, a lat and/or posterior-chain restriction is a part of the problem.[2] This means other factors (stiff muscles/tissues and/or joint restrictions) elsewhere in the body are contributing to poor overhead mobility.

The Wall Angel Screen
If you were able to look at a group of kids, most of these kids would be able to reach their arms overhead fully with ease. Whether it's playing on the handlebars at the jungle gym or climbing a tree, overhead mobility is rarely an issue! However, after years of sedentary lifestyle (sitting at a desk, reading, playing video games, staring at our phones), people develop poor posture.

Because of years of poor posture, the thoracic spine will stiffen and the pectoral muscles (major and minor) will adaptively shorten. The wall angel screening will show if you have any restrictions in gross overhead mobility.

To understand how the mobility of the thoracic spine and pecs affect overhead arm movement, try this simple test. Sit in a slouched position, with your upper back and shoulders rounded forward. Try to raise your arms as far as you can over your head. Now sit up as straight as possible with good posture and raise your arms again. Did you notice a difference?

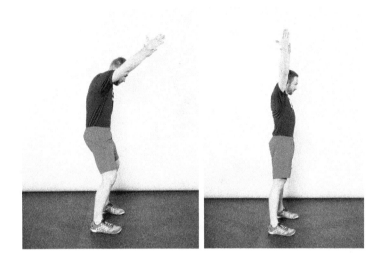

When you sit with good posture, you should be able to reach overhead much higher than sitting with crappy posture. You can also lift more weight with good posture.

To start the screening, find a wall and stand with your back to it. Your head and entire back should be in contact with the wall. Your feet should be four or five inches from the base.

Next, raise both of your arms to the side in an *L* position (as if you're making a football goal post with your arms). Without moving your head or lower back from the wall, try to flatten the back of your arms and hands against the wall. Don't let your lower back pop off the wall!

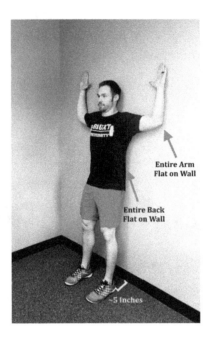

To pass, you must have your entire back flat against the wall. The elbows, forearms, and hands should be resting comfortably against the wall. Your head should also be in contact with the wall.

If you were unable to touch the entire wall with your arms, where did you feel the restriction? You may have felt tightness in your pecs, midback, or both. If so, you would benefit from upper-body mobility work, which we will discuss later. If you had pain at any time, seek the advice of a medical professional, as something more serious may need to be addressed. Don't be alarmed if you failed; this is a difficulty test to pass.

Final Thoughts

It's clear to see that many factors contribute to overhead mobility. If you can't move your arms into a good position overhead *without* a barbell, what do you think will happen when you try to perform an overhead squat or snatch? If you were unable to pass either of these screens, don't worry! Our goal is to highlight if you had any weak links in your upper body.

If you were able to pass both of these screens, congrats! This means you have good global upper-body mobility. You likely don't need to spend time stretching and mobilizing your upper body. I would recommend spending your valuable time on fixing any other issues that you have in the body.

9.2 Mobility Corner

I now want to share with you a few of my favorite mobility exercises to address any weak links you may have found in overhead mobility.

1. Mobilize (joint and soft tissue)
2. Stretch
3. Posterior-chain activation

Joint Mobilizations

A restriction in thoracic spine joint mobility should be the first thing to address. This type of stiffness will not always resolve with foam rolling or stretching. If you felt any tightness in your midback when trying to bring your arms to the wall during the wall angel screen, this tool should help!

One of the best tools to improve thoracic spine mobility

is to use a "peanut." Some manufactures make a fancy peanut, which will cost you a pretty dollar. However, you can save a lot of money by taping two tennis or two lacrosse balls together.

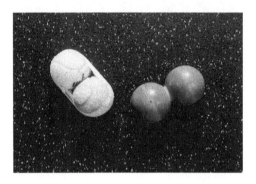

To perform a thoracic spine joint mobilization, lie on your back with your arms crossed in front of you. This will pull your shoulder blades (scapulas) "out" to the side. This will provide space to place the peanut. The tennis or lacrosse balls should rest on both sides of your spine.

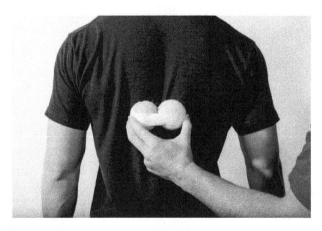

With your arms across your chest, perform a small crunch by raising your shoulders off the ground a few inches. Hold this position for a few seconds before returning to start position. Make sure not to hyper-extend your lower back during this movement. We want to only move from the midback.

The peanut acts as a fulcrum on the spine (much like the middle of a teeter-totter) during this movement. When this force is applied to a stiff joint, it can help improve mobility.

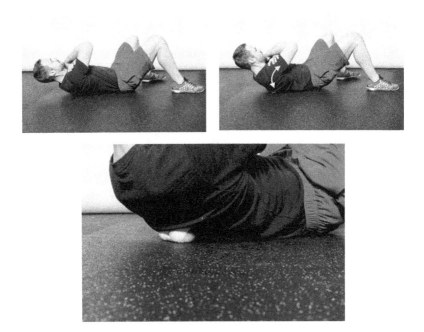

Perform two to three sets of fifteen repetitions on each segment of your midback that feels stiff.[3] If you don't feel any stiffness at a particular part of your spine during the movement, move the peanut up or down to another segment. It is normal to have restrictions in only a few of the thoracic spine joints.

You should not have intense pain during this maneuver. If you do, I recommend seeking out a medical professional such as a physical therapist or chiropractor.

Soft-Tissue Mobilization

Once joint restrictions have been addressed, the next step is to clear up any soft-tissue stiffness. We can do this with a foam roller and/or a lacrosse ball. Athletes with restricted lats and pecs need to be mobilizing on a daily basis!

To address the lats, start by lying on your side with one arm raised above your head. Work the foam roller into the large muscle on the outside of your armpit. This is where the lat muscle runs!

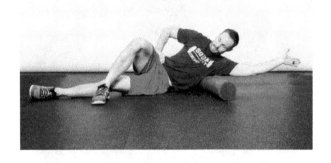

Move up and down this muscle until you find an area that may be tender. Pause on this spot for a few seconds before moving on. Do not move quickly during this drill! Instead, roll in a slow and rhythmical fashion.

To address the pecs, start by finding a wall. Trap a lacrosse or tennis ball between your chest and the wall. Move the ball around your muscle until you can find any tender areas. Perform slow movements with occasional pauses at each area.

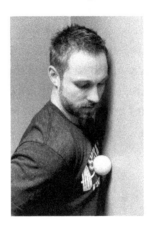

You can add in some active movement with this mobilization as well. Once you find a tender area, start moving your arm out to the side away from your body. This can add to the effectiveness of the exercise.

Stretch

Once soft-tissue mobilization is complete, the next step is stretching. I want to share with you my favorite stretches for enhancing overhead mobility.

1. Prayer stretch
2. Corner stretch
3. Foam-roller pec stretch

If you were unable to pass the supine lat-stretch screen, you would probably benefit from the prayer stretch. This is similar to the classic yoga pose called "child's pose."

Start in a kneeling position. Sit your hips back on your feet and push your hands out in front of you (one hand on top of the other). Next, let your chest drop down to the floor. Continue to reach with your arms together overhead while you let your breath out slowly. Try to sink your chest toward the ground. If you have stiffness in your lats, this should bring out a good stretch in your midback. I recommend holding this pose for thirty seconds.

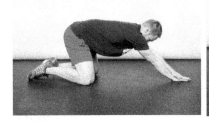
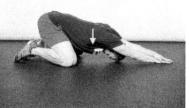

If you were unable to pass the wall angel screening, you would probably benefit from stretching the pec muscles (major and minor). Two easy stretches I use with my patients to clear up pec restrictions are the "corner stretch" and the "foam roller pec stretch."

Find a corner in the room you are in. Stand with your arms out to the side in an *L* position. Place your hands on the walls and slowly push into the corner. Make sure to keep your lower back from hyper-extending during this movement. You should feel a good stretch in your chest the more you push into the corner. This stretch has been shown in research to be one of the most efficient ways to elicit changes in pec minor muscle length.[3]

Be cautious not to push too hard with this stretch. Doing so can place harmful torque on your shoulder joints. The goal is to only feel this stretch in your pecs, not your shoulders. Hold this position for ten to thirty seconds.

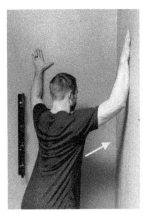 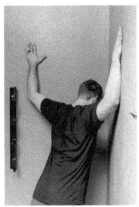

For some, the corner stretch can be too intense. The foam roller pec stretch is another good option. It is much easier to perform and places less torque on the shoulders.

Start by lying down with a foam roller positioned lengthwise along your back. The foam roller should rest in between your shoulder blades. Take a PVC pipe or a broomstick and raise your arms over your head as far as you can. Make sure to keep your entire back flat on the foam roller. You should feel a very light stretch in your chest as your arms hang in the air. The goal is to relax your upper body in this position and hold the low-load stretch for a long duration (about thirty seconds to one minute).

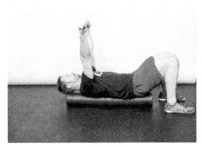 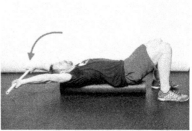

Do not perform this stretch with a barbell or any other heavy object in your hands. This can easily lead to too much torque on the shoulder joints. If you experience any tingling down your arms or in your hands, it's a sign you are stretching too aggressively.

Posterior-Chain Activation
After performing any of these upper-body drills, you need to strengthen the body into this newly gained mobility. It's easy to focus on mobility restrictions and forget about strengthening the muscles that maintain good posture! In my opinion, both are equally important in maintaining good overhead mobility.

If you had stiffness in your thoracic spine, you need to follow up your mobility work with some endurance exercises. To perform this, start by lying on your stomach with your arms in an *L* position out to the side. While focusing on your midback, perform a small chin tuck and lift your head off the ground. Hold this position while focusing on activating the muscles in between your shoulder blades for ten seconds.

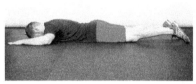 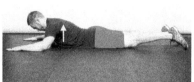

If you had flexibility problems in your lats or pecs, we also need to focus on activating the scapular stabilizers (posterior shoulder musculature and lower traps). This will be the topic of our next chapter!

Final Thoughts
After you have performed the corrective exercises, it's time to check and see the progress you have made. Remember to always use a test-retest strategy when performing mobility work.

Your overhead movement during the initial screenings should improve after performing these exercises. Mobility work should also lead to better technique in the overhead barbell movements. Checking both of these areas will allow you to see if the tools you are using are effective in addressing the change you desire.

The mobility exercises shared today are not magic pills for improving mobility. They will not fix any stiffness in one session. However, if you notice a small change in your movement quality with the test-retest method, we are on the right track.

Notes

1. G. Cook, L. Burton, K. Kiesel, G. Rose, and M. Bryant, *Movement: Functional Movement Systems. Screening Assessment Corrective Strategies* (Aptos, CA: On Target Publications, 2010).
2. K. D. Johnson and T. K. Grindstaff, "Thoracic Region Self-mobilization: A Clinical Suggestion," *International Federation of Sports Physical Therapy* 7, no. 2 (April 2012): 252–56.
3. J. D. Borstad and P. M. Ludewig, "Comparison of Three Stretches for the Pectoralis Minor Muscle," *Journal of Shoulder and Elbow Surgery* 15, no. 3 (May–June 2006): 324–30.

Chapter 10
The Stable Shoulder Blade

Imagine for a moment a young boy helping his father set up a tall ladder. The young boy kneels at the base of the ladder, firmly securing it to the ground. The father then pushes the ladder upward, leaning it against the side of their house.

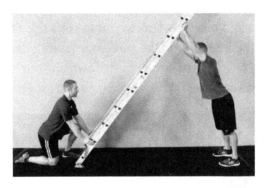

This illustration is precisely what happens at your shoulder every time you move your arm! The shoulder blade (scapula) acts just like the young boy in this story. The small muscles that attach and move the scapula help to "steer" your arm into place by keeping the base in a stable position.

The muscles of the upper back work together to maintain

the barbell in a good position during overhead barbell movements. Think what would happen if the father tried to set up the tall ladder without the help of his son to secure the base. This would be a recipe for disaster. The same scenario occurs when athletes perform overhead squats and snatches with poor scapular stability.

10.1 Screening for Scapular Instability

While there is a lot that goes into assessing your scapular stability, one simple test you can do at home is the *T* and *Y* screen. This is an easy way to uncover possible weak links in the muscles that secure your shoulder blade (seventeen to be exact).

Start by assuming a kneeling position with your chest facing the ground. Hold one arm directly out to your side (as if making one side of the letter *T*). Make sure your palm is facing toward the ground. Have a partner then push down on your outstretched arm for three seconds. Try to keep your arm from moving!

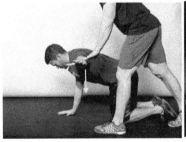
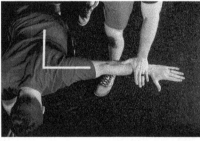

Next, take your outstretched arm and move it to an elevated position (as if now making one side of the letter *Y*). Again, have a partner push down on your outstretched arm for three seconds. Try to resist this movement as much as you can!

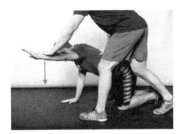 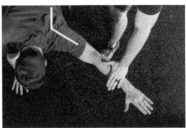

What did you feel? Was it easy or difficult for you to maintain your outstretched arm position? If you had a hard time keeping your arm from moving, it means you may have poor scapular stability.

Final Thoughts
Athletes who struggle with poor scapular stability often have difficulty with the overhead squat and barbell snatch movements. If left unchecked, this problem can even lead to the onset of shoulder and/or elbow pain. If you want to stay healthy and reach your true strength potential, focusing on stabilizing your scapula during overhead lifts is vital!

10.2 Corrective Exercise Corner
I now want to share with you two of my favorite corrective exercises to address overhead instability.

1. External rotation press
2. Kettle bell Turkish get-ups

Focus on your posture while performing each movement. An exercise performed with poor posture (i.e., rounded shoulders) only reinforces the problem we're trying to tackle. If you want to see any lasting improvements in your overhead stability, you *must* use good posture!

External Rotation Press
When athletes struggle to keep the barbell overhead during a snatch or overhead squat, they often allow the bar to fall forward. In order to fix this problem, we need to focus on activating the muscles that resist this forward collapse (the scapular stabilizers on the back of the shoulder).

Step 1: (Row) Grab a resistance band with your right hand. Pull the band toward you in a rowing motion. Your hand should finish directly in front of your elbow with your arm parallel to the ground. This engages the muscles that stabilize the shoulder blade.

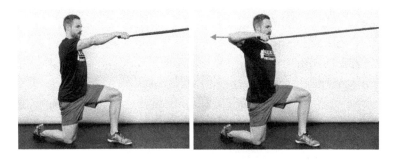

Step 2: (External rotation) From this position, rotate the shoulder backward. Your hand should now be facing the ceiling with your elbow bent to ninety degrees like an *L*.

Step 3: (Press) Next, push your hand overhead and hold for five seconds. The muscles that stabilize the shoulder blade should be working hard to keep your arm from falling forward.

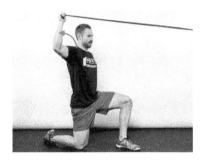 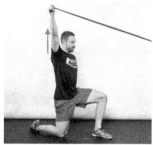

Step 4: Next, reverse the pattern and return to the start position. Lower the arm to the *L* position. Rotate forward until your arm is parallel to the ground. Finally, press your arm forward to end the movement.

Recommended Sets/Reps: ten repetitions of five-second holds in the overhead position for each arm.

Kettle Bell Turkish Get-Up
The get-up challenges the athlete to create scapular stability through a progression of movements. During each transition, every muscle that stabilizes the arm must work to keep the weight from falling forward.

Step 1: Start by lying on your back. Your left leg should be straight with your right knee bent. Hold a small weight with your right hand. Press the weight toward the ceiling.

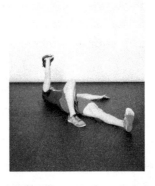

Step 2: Next, rotate your body onto your left side, propping yourself onto your elbow. Try to keep your left foot from coming off the ground during this transition. To maintain this position, think about forcing your left heel through the wall in front of you as you rotate.

Keep the weight from falling forward! To help with this, imagine yourself balancing a glass of water with the hand that is holding the weight. If your arm falls forward, the water will spill from the glass.

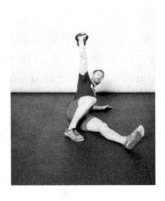

Step 3: Push yourself upward into a side plank. Pause during this transition and feel for the position of your scapula.

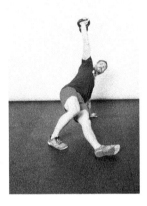

Step 4: Pull your left foot under your body and shift your weight onto your left knee. Pause again in this position for three seconds.

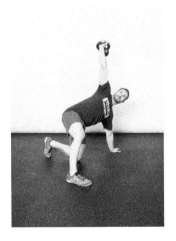

Step 5: Twist forward into a split kneeling position. Pause in this position for three seconds. Feel the muscles in the back of your shoulder working hard.

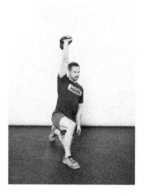

Step 6: Stand straight up, keeping your arm locked out above your head.

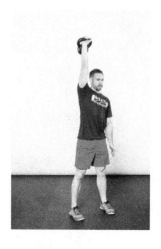

Step 7: To finish, reverse the same order of movements until you are lying again on the ground. To progress this exercise you can use a heavier kettle bell. You can also move to using a barbell for added difficulty.

Recommended Sets/Reps: three sets of ten repetitions.

Final Thoughts

If you want to perform overhead barbell lifts with good technique and without pain, it is vital that you improve and maintain good scapular stability.

Chapter 11
Debunking Squat Myths

11.1 Are Deep Squats Bad for Your Knees?

The squat is a staple exercise in almost every resistance-training program. Today, athletes of all ages and skill levels use the barbell squat to gain strength and power. However, a good amount of controversy still exists on its safety. There are many opinions when it comes to optimal squat depth. Some experts claim squatting as deep as possible (ass-to-grass) is the only way to perform the lift. Others believe deep squats are harmful to the knees and should never be performed. So who should we believe?

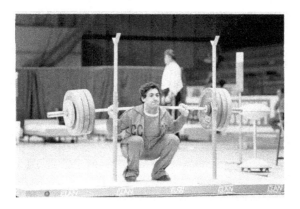

Used with permission from Bruce Klemens

History 101

To start, we need to discuss where the fear of deep squatting originated. Let's take a trip back to the 1950s. We can trace the safety concerns with the deep squat back to a man by the name of Dr. Karl Klein. The goal at that time was to understand the reason behind the rise in number of college football players sustaining serious knee injuries. He suspected these injuries were in part due to the use of full-range-of-motion deep squats during team weight training. Klein used a crude self-made instrument to analyze the knees of several weightlifters who frequently performed deep squats.

In 1961, he released his findings, stating that deep squatting stretched out the ligaments of the knee.[1] He claimed this was evidence that athletes who performed the deep squat were potentially compromising the stability of their knees and setting themselves up for injury. He went on to recommend that all squats be performed only to parallel depth.

Klein's theory was eventually picked up in a 1962 issue of *Sports Illustrated*. This was the catalyst he needed to spread the fear of deep squatting and save the knees of athletes everywhere. The American Medical Association (AMA) soon after came out with a position statement cautioning against the use of deep squats.[2] The Marine Corps eliminated the squat-jumper exercise from its physical-conditioning programs.[3] Even the superintendent for New York schools issued a statement banning gym teachers from using the full-depth squat in physical education classes.[4]

Some individuals disagreed with Dr. Klein. In May of 1964, Dr. John Pulskamp (a regular columnist in the notorious *Strength and Health*) wrote, "Full squats are not bad for the knees and they should certainly not be omitted out of fear of knee injury."[5] Despite Dr. Pulskamp's best efforts, the damage that Klein inflicted had been done. By the end of the decade, strength coaches across the country stopped teaching the full-depth squat. In some cases, the squat was dropped from training programs completely.[6]

Thanks to the advancements in exercise science and biomechanics research, we have learned so much more about forces sustained during squats. Let's now go over what we have learned in the past few decades in order to better understand what exactly happens at the knee joint during the deep squat.

Squatology 101

When we squat, our knees sustain two types of forces: shear and compressive. Shear forces are measured by how much the bones in our knee (femur and tibia) want to slide over each other in the opposite directions. These forces in high levels can be harmful to the ligaments inside the knee (ACL and PCL). These small ligaments are some of the primary structures that hold our knees together and limit excessive forward and backward movement.

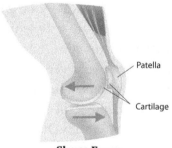

Shear Force

Compressive force is the amount of pressure from two parts of the body pushing on each other. Two different areas sustain this type of force in the knee. The meniscus absorbs the opposing stress between the tibia and the femur. The second type of compressive force is found between the backside of the patella (kneecap) and the femur. As the knee bends during the squat, the patella makes contact with the femur. The deeper the squat, the more connection between the patella and the femur.

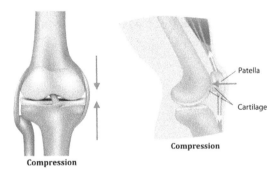

When we look at these forces (shear and compression), we see that they are typically inversely related. This means when the knee flexes during the squat, compressive forces increase while shear forces decrease.[7]

Ligament Safety

Some medical authorities have cautioned against the use of deep squats due to excessive strain placed on the ligaments. However, it appears these concerns are not based in science at all.

Science now tells us that the ligaments inside our knees are actually placed under very little stress in the bottom of a deep squat. The ACL (anterior cruciate ligament) is the most well-known ligament of the knee. ACL injuries are common in popular American sports such as football, basketball, soccer, lacrosse, and so forth. The stress to the ACL during a squat is actually highest during the first four inches of the squat descent (when the knee is bent around fifteen to thirty degrees).[8] As depth increases, the forces placed on the ACL significantly decrease. In fact, the highest forces ever measured on the ACL during a squat has only been found to be around 25 percent of its ultimate strength (the force needed to tear the ligament).[9]

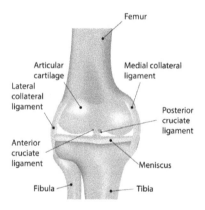

The PCL (posterior cruciate ligament) is the second ligament that is found inside the knee. During the squat, it sustains max forces just above a parallel squat position (around ninety degrees of knee flexion).[10] Just like the ACL, this ligament is never placed under excessive stress during the squat. The highest recorded forces on this ligament have been only 50 percent of the estimated strength in a young athlete's PCL.[11]

In fact, science has shown that the deeper you squat, the safer it is on the ligaments of your knee. Harmful shear forces are dramatically decreased due to an increase in compression. Also, the muscles in our legs work together to stabilize the knee. As we squat, the hamstrings work with the quadriceps to counteract and limit excessive movement deep inside the knee.[12]

Thus, the ACL and PCL stay unharmed no matter how deep the squat is!

Knee Stability
The original studies by Dr. Klein claimed squatting deep stretched out the ligaments that hold the knee together, ultimately leaving it unstable. However, these claims have never been replicated. Researchers have even used a copy of Klein's testing instrument in their own studies. Their findings disapproved Klein's research. They found that athletes who used the deep squat had no difference in the laxity of their knee ligaments than those who only squatted to parallel.[13]

Science has actually shown that squatting deep may have a protective effect on our knees by increasing their stability. In 1986, researchers compared knee stability among powerlifters, basketball players, and runners. After a heavy squat workout, the powerlifters actually had more stable knees than the basketball players (who just practiced for over an hour) and runners (who just ran ten kilometers) did. In 1989, another group of researchers were able to show that competitive weightlifters and powerlifters had knee ligaments that were less lax than those who never squatted.[15] Again and again, research has shown that the deep squat is a safe exercise to include in a healthy athlete's training program.

When Can Deep Squatting Be Harmful?

Theoretically, most of the damage that the knees would sustain from deep squats would be due to excessive compression forces. Some authorities claim that because deep squats raise compression forces at the knee, they cause the meniscus and the cartilage on the backside of the patella to wear away. While an increase in compression would lead to a greater susceptibility for injury, there has been no such cause-and-effect relationship established by science!

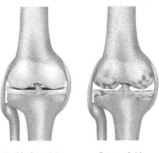

Healthy knee joint   Osteoarthritis

If this were true, we would expect to see extreme amounts of arthritis in the knees of weightlifters and powerlifters. Fortunately, this is not the case. There is little evidence of cartilage wear in the knees because of long-term weight training. In fact, elite weightlifters and powerlifters (who sustain loads up to six times bodyweight to the knee in the bottom of a deep squat) have relatively healthy knees compared to you and me![16]

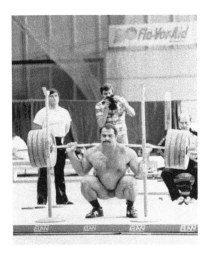

Used with permission from Bruce Klemens

Considerations for Squatting Deep

Every coach must consider a few things when determining optimal squat depth for an athlete. Everyone should have the capability to perform a bodyweight squat to full depth, period. That being said, the depth of the barbell squat should be based on the requirements of an athlete's sport. A weightlifter, for example, needs to establish strength in the full-depth squat in order to lift the most amount of weight on the competition platform. On the other hand, a barbell ass-to-grass squat is not necessary for a soccer player. He or she can still gain efficient strength and power from a parallel-depth squat.

The injury history of the athlete also needs to be taken into account when determining optimal squat depth. Often athletes will ignore pain in their pursuit of performance gains. The phrases "no pain, no gain" and "know the difference between hurt and injured" cannot apply to the weight room. Pain is like the warning light in a car. The light is indicating something is wrong. Just as ignoring your car's warning light will lead to engine problems, pushing through pain in the weight room will lead to injury of the physical body. For this reason, if an athlete is injured and has knee pain, deep squats may not be the best choice. The depth of the squat must be limited to a pain-free range if we want to stay healthy and continue to compete injury free.

Squat depth should also be limited if it cannot be performed with good technique. Poor movement only increases our risk for injury. An athlete's body is like a finely tuned sports car. Constantly driving pedal to the metal and taking aggressive turns will lead the car to break down faster. The same goes for squatting. You can only lift so much weight poorly for so long before your body sustains an injury. Squatting to full depth poorly is a great way to invite injury.

So what have we found out since 1964? Contrary to mainstream belief, we now know that squatting deep or "ass-to-grass" is actually not as dangerous as Dr. Klein made it out to be. Research again and again has failed to support the theory that deep squats are bad for the knees in healthy athletes.

For athletes with healthy knees, performing the squat to full depth should not cause injury as long as heavy loads are not used excessively. Proper training programs should employ light, medium, and heavy intensity cycles throughout the year in order to lessen any harmful effects of constant heavy loading. Now that you have a deeper understanding of full-depth squats, feel free to get that ass to the grass!

11.2 Should My Knees Go Past My Toes?

There is a strongly held belief by many that the knees should never go over the toes when squatting. I was recently guest lecturing to a class of physical therapy students at the University of Missouri. I asked a simple question. "How many people here think we should never have our knees go past the toes while squatting?" Following my inquiry, every single student held up his or her hand. The next thing I said was, "You're all wrong."

No one is certain where this myth started. However, it has become a mainstay in today's fitness and medical worlds. The instruction is even a part of the National Strength and Conditioning Association's (NSCA) guidelines for how to teach a proper squat.[12]

Yet, is it really all that dangerous? Since 2005, I have had the opportunity to watch and compete on the same platform with some of the best weightlifters in the United States. To lift the most amount of weight during the clean, a weightlifter must catch the barbell in a deep-squat position. In order to remain upright with the bar secured on the chest, the knees of many lifters will move past their toes. Are these weightlifters putting their knees in harm's way every time they lift the barbell?

Knees Over Toes?
The cue to limit the knees from moving past the toes during the squat is really nothing more than a quick fix to a deeper problem. In hindsight, the originators of the cue were likely well-intentioned strength coaches or physical therapists.

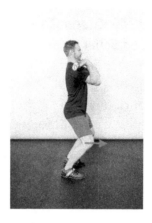

When athletes squat poorly, they often move from their ankles first. As the ankles move, it causes the knees to hinge forward. The weight of the body is then shifted forward on to the balls of the feet. This type of movement problem has been called the "knees-first" approach. Moving in this way leads to greater shear forces on the knee joint and contributes to increased risk of injury and eventually to pain.[4]

To many individuals, this issue would appear to be a problem of the knee. Athletes who squat poorly by moving their knees forward often develop pain. Therefore, limiting this forward movement solves the problem...right? However, limiting the knees from moving only addresses the symptoms of a bigger problem.

The issue is actually with balance. The knee is only a hinge joint. It will only move forward based on what goes on at the ankle and hip. Instead of focusing so much on what is going on at the knee, we should really be focusing on the hip and ankle joint when we squat.

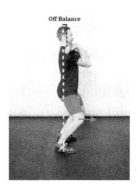

Off Balance

One of the absolutes of squatting is that our center of gravity must remain over the middle of our feet. This allows our body to remain balanced and work efficiently to produce strength and power. During a bodyweight squat, our center of gravity is located around our belly button. During weight training, the barbell becomes our center of gravity. The efficiency of our movement is dictated by how well we can maintain this weight over the middle of our feet.

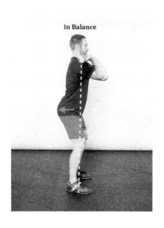

In Balance

When the knees hinge forward early in the squat, the athlete's center of gravity is shifted forward onto the balls of his or her feet. Therefore, the cue to limit the knees from moving forward is actually correcting for a weight-shift problem. It has little to do with the knee joint itself and more to do with ensuring that the athlete stays balanced.

Sitting Back in the Squat

So how do we correct for moving from the ankles first? The cue to "sit back" or to "push the hips back" allows the athlete to move from his or her hips first instead of his or her ankles during the descent of the squat. This engages the powerhouse of the body (the posterior chain). Doing so also limits premature forward movement of the knees. This allows the athlete's center of gravity to remain over the middle of the foot.

However, the cue to limit the knees from moving forward only works to a point. In order to reach full depth in the squat, there comes a time when the knees must eventually move forward. The deeper we squat, the more our knees will have to move forward in order to remain balanced. This concept can be hard to understand for many in the medical community. Let me explain.

In order to reach full depth in the squat, the hips must eventually be pulled under the torso. This allows us to remain balanced and keep our chest upright. Because the knee is a hinge joint that moves based on what happens at the hip and ankle, it will be forced forward at this point.

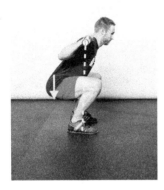 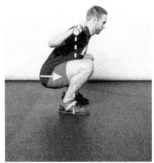

It is very normal for athletes to have their knees move forward even past their toes. It all comes down to weight distribution and the ability to maintain their center of gravity over the middle of the foot.

We should be concerned about *when* the knees more forward past the toes, not *if*.

The Barbell Squats
In the sport of powerlifting, athletes will commonly use a low-bar back squat technique. This position secures the bar farther down on the back over the middle of the shoulder blade (scapula). The athlete will use the "hips back" approach during the squat with an inclined trunk position in order for the bar to remain balanced over the middle of the feet. This allows the majority of the weight to be hoisted through the strength of the

hips and minimal forward movement of the knees.[13] Because our hips are extremely strong, athletes use this technique to lift over one thousand pounds!

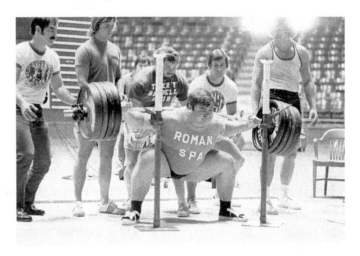

Used with permission from Bruce Klemens

However, this squat technique can only descend to a certain point. If an "ass-to-grass" squat were to be attempted with the low-bar back squat, the athlete would eventually fold in half like an accordion!

In the sport of weightlifting, athletes commonly use the high-bar back squat, front squat, and overhead squat techniques. These barbell movements resemble the positions an athlete will use during the competition lifts of the snatch and clean and jerk. These lifts require a more balanced approach between the hips and knees in order to maintain an upright trunk. Athletes must descend as deep as possible in order to effectively lift tremendous weights.

By allowing the knees to eventually move forward, the weightlifter can descend into a deep clean or snatch without falling forward. For this reason, the weightlifter cannot perform the front squat like the low-bar technique of the powerlifter.

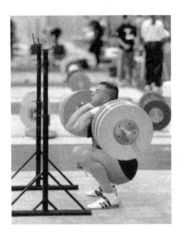

Used with permission from Bruce Klemens

While shear forces have been shown to increase in the deep-squat position with forward knees, the body can handle them appropriately without risk for injury.[14] If done properly with a "hip-first" approach, the knees going past the toes is not only safe but necessary.

Take Away
The next time you watch someone squat, focus on which joint moves first. Someone who moves poorly will move with a "knees-first" approach. On the other hand, an athlete who moves with good technique will move with the hips back first.

Science has shown that the knees of healthy athletes are relatively safe in the bottom of a deep squat.[4,14] There is no denying this research. As long as excessive loading is limited and good technique is used, the knees *can* and *must* move past the toes in the bottom of a squat in order to allow the hips to drop fully.

Strength coach Michael Boyle once wrote, "The question is not where does the knee go, as much as where is the weight distributed and what joint moves first?"[15] Remember, the knee is only a hinge joint. As long as it is kept stable (in line with the feet), we should not worry about it. Proper squatting is all about moving at the hips first and staying balanced. The rest takes care of itself.

11.3 Toes Forward or Angled Out?

During a recent Squat University seminar, I was approached by an athlete who wondered why I had asked everyone to show me his or her squat with his or her toes straightforward. This was definitely not the first time I've been asked this question. There's a lot of controversy in the fitness world today when it comes to recommended foot position during the squat. Some experts say our feet should be straightforward all the time. Others advocate the toes should turn out at an angle. So who is correct?

This is actually a trick question. The answer is both. Let me explain.

Argument for Toes Forward

The squat is a movement first and an exercise second. When I screen a new athlete, I want to see his or her ability to squat with shoes off and toes facing forward. My goal is to assess his or her *movement*. This method allows me to see any weak links with the athlete.

Squatting with your feet straightforward is more difficult than with the toes pointed slightly outward. I don't think many would argue with that notion. **However, that is the point of the screen.**

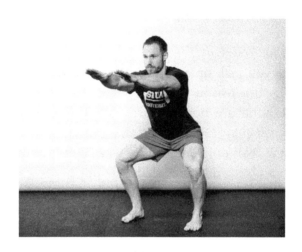

In order to squat to full depth with the toes straightforward, athletes must have adequate ankle and hip mobility and sufficient pelvic/core control. They must also have acceptable coordination and balance. Turning the toes out at an angle allows a majority of people to achieve a full-depth squat with a more upright chest position. A few individuals will always simply be unable to get into a deep-squat position due to abnormal anatomical reasons. Some people are born with genetic abnormalities. With that said, most athletes should be able to reach ass-to-grass with a squat.

The bodyweight squat sets the movement foundation for other athletic actions such as jumping and landing. Many knee injuries occur when you land with your foot pointing out and the knee caving in. Players who have to jump and cut will tear their ACL when the knee caves in and rotates. My goal is for athletes to land and jump with good mechanics, therefore decreasing their lack of season-ending injuries.

Argument for Toes Out

As soon as you pick up a barbell, the squat now becomes an exercise. For this reason, there are slight changes in the movement pattern that are more sport specific. This includes turning the toes out *slightly*. Doing so creates a mechanical advantage for the squat. Not only does it give us a slightly wider base of support, but also it does not challenge our pelvic control and mobility to the fullest extent.[19]

This is why some athletes can squat deeper when they turn their toes out. By externally rotating the hips, we can usually achieve a deeper and better-looking squat.

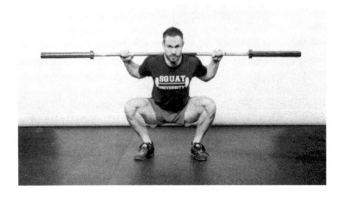

When our hips externally rotate, the adductor muscles on the inside of our legs are lengthened. As we squat, these muscles are put in a better position to produce force (length-tension relationship). This simply means the adductors are turned on and recruited to a greater degree during the squat if you turn your toes out slightly.[17] The adductor magnus specifically has been shown to help produce hip extension (the action of standing up from a squat).[18] More help from the adductors means a stronger and more efficient way to move the barbell.

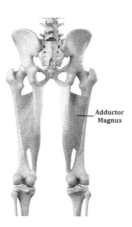

Turning the toes out, however, only changes the activation of the adductor muscle group. The glutes and quads (the main movers in the squat) are not significantly activated to a greater extent.[16] Research has shown that turning the toes out more than thirty degrees is less effective.[17] For this reason, you should perform barbell squats with your feet turned out anywhere from ten to thirty degrees. Always use a position that is most comfortable for your body. Remember, no two squats will look exactly the same. It's normal and expected for you and your friend to have different squat stances while lifting the barbell.

Final Thoughts
The argument is simple. I believe we should have the capability to perform a bodyweight squat with the toes relatively straightforward. If you cannot, more than likely you need to work on some things. I recommend turning your toes out when you squat with a barbell for optimal performance.

This is the difference between training and screening. Screening should point out and illuminate limitations in how we move. Training should reinforce and strengthen our current movement capabilities. When coaching athletes, it's your job to know the difference between screening and training.

Notes

1. T. Todd, "Historical Opinion: Karl Klein and the Squat," *National Strength and Conditioning Association Journal* 6, no. 3 (June–July 1984): 26–67.
2. J. Underwood, "The Knee Is Not for Bending," *Sports Illustrated* 16 (1962): 50.
3. J. R. Pulskamp, "Ask the Doctor," *Strength and Health* (May 1964): 82.
4. B. J. Schoenfeld, "Squatting Kinematics and Kinetics and Their Application to Exercise Performance," *Journal of Strength and Conditioning Research* 24, no. 12 (2010): 3497–506.
5. G. Li, S. Zayontx, E. Most, L. E. DeFrante, J. F. Suggs, and H. E. Rubash, "Kinematics of the Knee at High Flexion Angles: An In Vitro Investigation," *Journal of Orthopedic Research* 27, no. 6 (2004): 699–706.
6. J. C. Gullett, M. D. Tillman, G. M. Gutierrez, and J. W. Chow, "A Biomechanical Comparison of Back and Front Squats in Healthy Trained Individuals," *Journal of Strength and Conditioning Research* 23 (2009): 284–92.
7. R. F. Escamilla, G. F. Fleisig, N. Zheng, J. E. Lander, S. W. Barrentine, et al., "Effects of Technique Variations on Knee Biomechanics during the Squat and Leg Press," *Medicine and Science in Sports Exercise* 33, no. 9 (2001): 1552–66.
8. E. Myers, "Effect of Selected Exercise Variables on Ligament Stability and Flexibility of the Knee," *Research Quarterly* 42, no. 4 (1971): 411–22.

9. M. E. Steiner, W. A. Grana, K. Chillag, and E. Schelberg-Karnes, "The Effect of Exercise on Anterior-Posterior Knee Laxity," *American Journal of Sports Medicine* 14, no. 1 (1986): 24–29.
10. T. Chandler, G. Wilson, and M. Stone, "The Effect of the Squat Exercise on Knee Stability," *Medicine and Science in Sports Exercise* 21, no. 3 (1989): 299–303.
11. B. Fitzgerald and G. R. McLatachie, "Degenerative Joint Disease in Weight-Lifters Fact or Fiction," *British Journal of Sports Medicine* 14, no. 2 & 3 (August 14, 1980): 97–101.
12. R. W. Earle and T. R. Baechle, *Essentials of Strength Training and Conditioning* (Champaign, IL: Human Kinetics, 2008), 250–351.
13. P. A. Swinton, R. Lloyd, J. W. L. Keogh, et al., "A Biomechanical Comparison of the Traditional Squat, Powerlifting Squat, and Box Squat," *Journal of Strength and Conditioning Research* 26, no. 7 (2012): 1805–16.
14. H. Hartman, K. Wirth, and M. Klusemann, "Analysis of the Load on the Knee Joint and Vertebral Column with Changes in Squatting Depth and Weight Load," *Sports Medicine* 43, no. 10 (2013): 993–1008.
15. M. Boyle, "Knees Over Toes?" accessed January 25, 2016, Strengthcoach.com.
16. D. R. Clark, M. I. Lambert, and A. M. Hunter, "Muscle Activation in the Loaded Free Barbell Squat: A Brief Review," *Journal of Strength and Conditioning Research* 26, no. 4 (2012): 1169–78.

17. G. R. Pereira, G. Leporace, D. D. V. Chagas, et al., "Influence of Hip External Rotation on Hip Adductor and Rectus Femoris Myoelectric Activity During a Dynamic Parallel Squat," *Journal of Strength and Conditioning Research* 24, no. 10 (2010): 2749–52.
18. W. F. Dostal, G. L. Soderberg, and J. G. Andrews, "Actions of Hip Muscles," *Physical Therapy Journal* 66, no. 3 (1986): 351–59.
19. G. Cook, L. Burton, K. Kiesel, G. Rose, and M. Bryant, *Movement: Functional Movement Systems. Screening Assessment Corrective Strategies* (Aptos, CA: On Target Publications, 2010).

Photo Attribution
1. Compression Anterior View: AlilaMedicalMedia/Shutterstock.com
2. Compression Lateral View: AlilaMedicalMedia/Shutterstock.com
3. Shear Force: AlilaMedicalMedia/Shutterstock.com
4. Ligaments of Knee: Joshya/Shutterstock.com
5. Osteoarthritis: AlilaMedicalMedia/Shutterstock.com
6. Adductor Magnus: SebastianKaulitzki/Shutterstockc.com

Chapter 12
The Real Science of the Squat

Why is front squatting more difficult than back squatting when using the same weight? Is the low-bar back squat better for your knees than the high-bar variation? These are all common questions some of us have. In order to answer these questions, we have to look behind the curtain of movement and understand the science of squatting.

If you're a car person, you probably want to know exactly how your engine works. You've probably read articles describing the differences between the Chevy Corvette and the Ford Mustang. You understand how horsepower and torque production are different between a turbocharged V6 engine versus a standard V8.

This is your introductory class for the mechanics of the body. We will discuss the differences in torque generations between the squat techniques, as well as what that means for your training. As a word of caution: This chapter can be a little difficult to comprehend. However, I will do my best to teach these concepts as simply as possible. Welcome to Squat Biomechanics 101.

12.1 Squat Biomechanics

The term *biomechanics* simply refers to the study of forces and to how they act on the human body. Biomechanics is the science of breaking down the way we move.

When sport scientists analyze athletes, they often investigate the different forces that are produced during movement. Torque is one of the different parameters that are studied. Torque is the force that causes rotation around a joint.

To explain what torque is and how it affects our body, I like to use a simple illustration that I first learned in my college physics class. Many strength and conditioning professionals have used similar examples in their teachings. In particular, Mark Rippitoe's work in his book *Starting Strength* along with the research from Professor Andrew Fry are two great examples that are worth reading.[1,2]

Try holding a dumbbell in front of yourself at shoulder height. Do you feel the weight of the dumbbell trying to pull your arm down? What you're feeling is the force of gravity. It always pulls straight down. As gravity pulls down on the dumbbell, it causes a rotational force at the shoulder joint. This force is torque. The muscles of the shoulder must then be activated to overcome this force in order to keep the weight from moving.

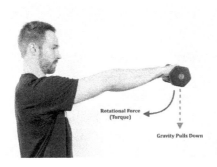

In order to calculate how much torque is generated at the shoulder, we need to know a few things. First, we need to find the length of the person's arm holding the weight. This length between the point of rotation (the shoulder in this case) and the line of force acting upon that joint (the pull of gravity) creates what we call a lever arm.

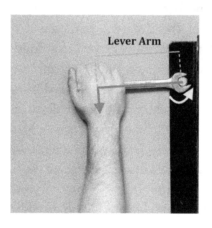

You can also think of the lever arm as a wrench turning a bolt. When the wrench is pulled down, it creates the rotational force torque that turns the bolt.

Let's take a trip back to physics class and discover how we can calculate this rotational force at a joint. A simple equation to write down is:

$$\text{Torque} = \text{Moment arm} \times \text{force}$$

You'll notice the word *moment arm* in the equation instead of lever arm. The moment arm is the perpendicular distance from the start of the lever arm (joint axis) to the vertical force of gravity. It always runs at ninety degrees. For this reason, it will change in length based on the angle the lever arm is held.

In our example, the arm is being held straight out in front of the body. This means the arm is already perpendicular to the vertical force of gravity. For this reason, the length of our arm (lever arm) will be the exact length of the moment arm. Let's assume your arm is about seventy-five centimeters in length (roughly thirty inches). Yes, most mathematical equations also use the metric system.

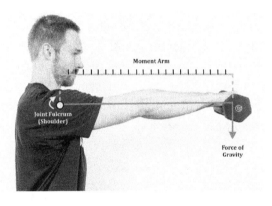

In order to calculate torque, we also need to know how much force is acting on the lever arm. Let's assume the dumbbell weighs ten pounds; now convert that ten pounds to 44.5 newtons (the unit for force). To get 44.5 newtons, you must convert ten pounds to 4.54 kilograms. This is then multiplied by 9.8 m/s^2 (standard gravity acceleration), resulting in 44.5 newtons. A heavier weight would therefore lead to more newtons of force.

The equation for torque at the shoulder would look something like this.

Torque = moment arm × force
   = 0.75 meters × 44.5 newtons
   = 33.4 NM or newton meters of force
      acting upon the shoulder

This means the muscles of our shoulder need to overcome 33.4 newton meters of force (roughly 24.6 foot-pounds of force) to lift the ten-pound weight past the extended position straight out from the body.

You may be asking yourself, "What happens if I raise my arm to a different position?" If we raise the dumbbell above our shoulder joint, we change the length of the moment arm. This is because the arm is no longer perpendicular to the vertical force of gravity. While the length of our arm (the lever) is still the same, the moment arm is now shorter than when our arm was extended straight in front of us.

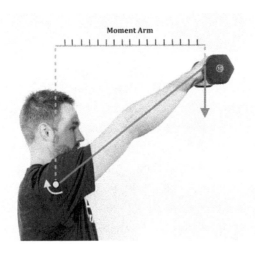

This decrease in moment arm length changes the torque placed on the shoulder joint. Let's assume we lifted the arm to an angle of 130 degrees. Because we don't know the new moment arm length, we need to use trigonometry to calculate this distance. The equation for torque at the shoulder would look something like this.

$$\text{Torque} = (\text{moment arm} \times \sin\Theta)(\text{force})$$
$$= (0.75 \text{ meters} \times \sin 130°)(44.5 \text{ newtons})$$
$$= 25.4 \text{ NM or newton meters}$$

When the arm is raised to the higher position, the moment arm becomes shorter. The dumbbell is creating less torque on the shoulder joint. This is why it's easier to hold the dumbbell close to your chest rather than straight out in front of you.

Another easy way to understand this concept is to perform a slow forward punch with the dumbbell. Is it harder or easier to hold the dumbbell away from your body? Obviously, the weight is easier to hold when it's close to your body! That's because the moment arm (from weight to shoulder joint) is shorter in this position. A small moment arm generates less torque on a joint when lifting a weight.

12.2 Squat Analysis 1.0

When we look at the squat, we typically look at three main areas:

1. The knee joint
2. The hip joint
3. The lower back

We need to know two things when trying to calculate the forces at these joints during the squat. First, we need to know the position or angle of the joints. To measure torque, a freeze-frame or snapshot of the moving body is often taken. This allows us to calculate how much torque is being generated at a specific moment in time. This is called a static model.[3]

While the static model for determining joint torques isn't perfect, most experts suggest that it still yields results within 10 percent of true torque values.[4]

When the squat is paused in a certain position, we can then measure the angle of the joints. The back angle is formed by an imaginary connection between the trunk and the floor. The hip angle is formed by the position of the back and the thigh. The knee angle is formed by the thigh and the position of the lower leg.

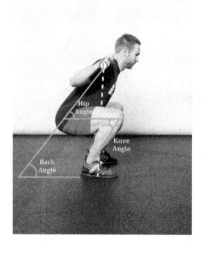

Breakout Tip: The knee angle is measured at the point of rotation (knee joint). When the leg is straight, the knee is in zero degrees of flexion. As the knee moves into a flexed position (like when we squat), the angle increases. This is why a deep-squat position will be recorded as a knee angle of greater than 120 degrees instead of sixty degrees.

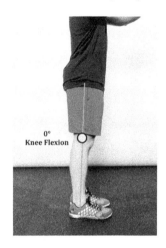
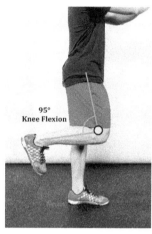

Next, we need to measure the length of the lever arms. These distances will change based on the anatomy of the athlete and what kind of barbell squat technique he or she is performing.

During the squat, gravity pulls down on the barbell just as it did with the dumbbell from our previous illustration. Gravity is often represented as a vertical line drawn through the middle of the barbell. This vertical line then runs through the body and divides the thigh.

During the squat, the barbell should track vertically over the middle of an athlete's foot. We can use this imaginary line to represent the vertical pull of gravity.

The distance from this vertical line to the center of the joint becomes a lever. Just like the wrench turning the bolt, the length of the lever arm can help us determine the length of the moment arm.[5] The longer the moment arm, the more torque that will be generated at that joint during the squat.

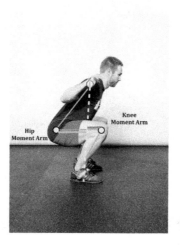

Often sport scientists will analyze the squat at a parallel squat position (hip crease in line with the knee).[6, 7] At this position (just like the athlete holding the dumbbell directly in front of the body), the lever arm and moment arm will be the same length.

High-Bar Back Squat Analysis (225 pounds)
Let's say we have an athlete squat 225 pounds (102 kilograms) with a high-bar back-squat technique. This technique places the bar on top of the shoulders and upper trapezius muscles near the base of the neck. It is commonly used by weightlifters as it

closely mimics the positions used in the competition lifts of the snatch and clean.

At the parallel position of this squat, we can freeze-frame the movement. For this illustration, let's say the knee ends up at an angle of 125 degrees and the angle of the hip is fifty-five degrees. The back angle would also be fifty-five degrees. Since we are assuming a parallel thigh position to the floor, the hip angle and back angle will be the same.

In order to simplify this analysis (and save ourselves some difficult trigonometry), we're going to measure the moment arms. Assume the knee moment arm in this high-bar back squat is 7.5 inches long (or 0.19 meters for mathematical purposes) and the hip moment arm is 10.5 inches long (or 0.27 meters). Remember, the moment arm length is the perpendicular distance from the joint to the vertical line of gravity that runs through the middle of the leg. This means the overall thigh length is eighteen inches long (hip lever arm + knee lever arm = full thigh length).

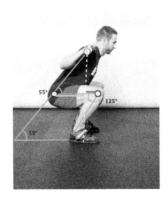

For the purposes of this analysis, the lower back will be represented as the connection of the spine to the pelvis. For this reason, the moment arm will be the distance from this point to the vertical line of gravity. Because this axis of rotation is relatively close to the hip joint, the back lever arm will be exactly the same distance as the hip lever arm.[1]

In order to do this calculation, we also need to figure in the weight of the barbell so we know how much force is pulling down. The weight of 225 pounds is equal to 1,000.85 newtons of force. We can now plug these numbers into our mathematical equation to determine torque.

Torque = moment arm × force
= 0.19 meters × 1,000.85 newtons
= 190.2 NM or newton meters of force acting upon the knee joint at 125°

Torque = moment arm × force
= 0.27 meters × 1,000.85 newtons
= 270 NM or newton meters of force acting upon the hip joint and lumbar/pelvis complex at 55°

Low-Bar Back Squat Analysis (225 pounds)

What if this same athlete now squatted 225 pounds with a different technique? Let's assume this athlete is now lifting with a low-bar back-squat technique. This variation uses a bar position that is two to three inches lower on the back than the high-bar back-squat technique. The bar commonly rests in the middle of the shoulder blade. Powerlifters commonly use it as it enables them to lift heavier weights.[5] In order to maintain balance (bar positioned over the middle of the feet), the chest must lean forward to a greater degree.[6]

Doing so does two things to the mechanical levers of the body. First, the forward lean of the trunk drives the hips backward. This lengthens the hip and back moment arm. It also shortens the knee moment arm.

Let's assume the knee moment arm is now 5.5 inches (0.14 meters) compared to the 7.5 inches during the high-bar technique. This would obviously lengthen the hip moment arm from 10.5 inches to 12.5 inches (0.32 meters).

At the parallel freeze-frame position, we see this lifter assuming a slightly different position.

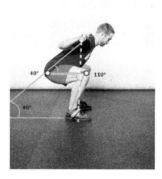

- Knee angle of 110 degrees (larger or more open than the high-bar technique)
- Hip and back angle of forty degrees (a smaller or more closed angle than the high-bar technique due to the more inclined chest position)

Torque = moment arm × force
 = 0.14 meters × 1,000.85 newtons
 = 140.1 NM or newton meters of force acting upon the knee joint at 110°

Torque = moment arm × force
 = 0.32 meters × 1,000.85 newtons
 = 320.3 NM or newton meters of force acting upon the hip joint and lumbar/pelvis complex at 40°

Front Squat Analysis (225 pounds)

Let's now look at the front squat. The front squat loads the joints differently than the previous two techniques. This is because the bar is held on the chest. This will require a more vertical trunk position in order to keep the bar positioned over the middle of the foot and allow the body to remain in balance. This lift is also used often by weightlifters as the movement closely mimics the clean movement.

The hips and knees will inevitably be pushed forward in order to maintain balance because the trunk must be held in a more upright position. If you try to front squat and push your hips back too far, the bar will likely roll off your chest and end up on the ground.

Let's assume the athlete's knee moment arm length is now 8.5 inches (0.22 meters). This is longer than the high-bar back squat. This is a common change as the knee frequently translates a bit farther forward in the front squat in order to remain in balance. This longer knee moment arm then creates a shorter hip moment arm, now measured at 9.5 inches (0.24 meters).

If we freeze-frame the front squat in the parallel thigh position, we see a few differences compared to the other squats.

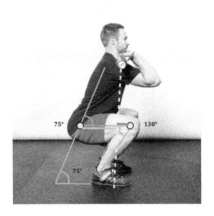

- Knee angle of 130 degrees (smaller or more closed compared to both back-squat techniques due to the more forward knee position)
- Hip and back angles of seventy-five degrees (larger or more open compared to the back-squat techniques due to the more upright chest position)

Torque = moment arm × force
       = 0.22 meters × 1,000.85 newtons
       = 220.2 NM or newton meters of force acting upon the knee joint at 130°

Torque = moment arm × force
= 0.24 meters × 1,000.85 newtons
= 240.2 NM or newton meters of force acting upon the hip joint and lumbar/pelvis complex at 75°

Comparative Analysis (225 pounds)

In this chapter, we assessed an athlete lifting a barbell loaded to 225 pounds (102 kilograms) with three squat technique variations. After calculating torque at the same depth across all three squats, we are able to see a few interesting things:

- The front squat placed the most amount of torque on the knee joint (220.2 newton meters) followed closely by the high-bar back squat (190.2 newton meters) and then by the low-bar back squat (140.1 newton meters). This means the front squat placed roughly 15 percent more torque on the knees than the high-bar squat and 57 percent more than the low-bar squat.
- The front squat placed less torque on the hip and lower back (240.2 newton meters at the lumbar/pelvis connection) compared to both back squat techniques (high-bar 270 newton meters and low-bar 320.3 newton meters). This means the front squat placed 12 percent less torque on the hip than the high-bar back squat and 25 percent less than the low-bar back squat.

If an athlete lifts the same weight with all three squat techniques, we can assume the front squat will be the most difficult to perform. According to this analysis, the low-bar back squat would be the easiest and most efficient way to lift the 225 pounds. The low-bar back squat is the most mechanically efficient technique. It all comes down to leverage. Mechanically, our bodies can squat more weight when the moment arm is longest at the hips.[5]

Many experienced lifters will agree that it's easier to lift more weight with the back-squat technique when compared to the front squat. Also, when watching a powerlifting meet, almost all of the lifters will use a low-bar back squat to compete and not the high-bar squat.

12.3 Squat Analysis 2.0

We now need to take a deeper look at the three squat techniques and compare them realistically. In the first section of this chapter, we didn't discuss what happens when the pull on the lever changes. Torque can be manipulated by not only changing the length of the moment arm but also by changing the amount of force pulling down on the lever.

When holding a ten-pound dumbbell out in front of your shoulder, there is roughly 44.5 newtons of force pulling down on your joint. This value represents the force of gravity's acceleration acting upon the weight. In our illustration, this created 33.4 newton meters of torque at the shoulder joint. We came to this number by plugging in the length of the moment arm (0.75 meters or roughly thirty inches), the angle of the arm, and the weight of the dumbbell.

The equation for torque at the shoulder looks something like this.

Torque = moment arm × force
= 0.75 meters × 44.5 newtons
= 33.4 NM or newton meters of force acting upon the shoulder

On the other hand, what if we now picked up a twenty-pound dumbbell and tried to raise and hold it at the same extended position? This weight would then be converted to about eighty-nine newtons of force. To get eighty-nine newtons, you must convert twenty pounds to 9.1 kilograms. This is then multiplied by 9.8 m/s^2 (standard gravity acceleration) to end up with eighty-nine newtons. If we assume the length of our arm didn't change, the mathematical equation to calculate the new torque value would be:

Torque = moment arm × force
= 0.75 meters × 89 newtons
= 66.75 NM or newton meters of force acting upon the shoulder

Now that we know how torque can be manipulated by changing either the moment arm length and/or the amount of force pulling down on the lever, let's now analyze the squat with weights that are more natural to each lift. A conservative estimate would be that an athlete could squat 15 percent more weight using a low-bar technique when compared to the high-bar technique. Most powerlifters use the low-bar variation over a high-bar back squat in competition for this reason. We could also make an educated guess and say most athletes could squat 15 percent more in the high-bar back squat compared to the front squat.

If we assume a one-repetition maximum in the low-bar back squat to be five hundred pounds, this would mean this individual could theoretically high-bar back squat 435 pounds and front squat around 378 pounds. Let's see how the change in weight on the barbell changes the torque placed on the various joint complexes of the body.

Low-Bar Back Squat (five hundred pounds)
If we assume a lifter is capable of a five-hundred-pound low-bar back squat, this means there will be 2,224.11 newtons of force now pulling down on the bar. This is a much larger value than we saw with the previous 225-pound loaded barbell.

For this analysis, we will use the exact same lever arm lengths and joint positions from the previous illustration. We'll again freeze-frame the squat at the parallel position (hip crease in line with the knee).[4] The only thing that we'll change will be the weight on the bar.

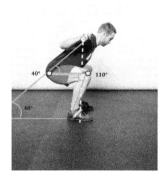

Torque = moment arm × force
 = 0.14 meters × 2,224.11 newtons
 = 311.4 NM or newton meters of force acting upon the knee joint at 110°

Torque = moment arm × force
 = 0.32 meters × 2,224.11 newtons
 = 711.7 NM or newton meters of force acting upon the hip joint and lumbar/pelvis complex at 40°

High-Bar Back Squat Analysis (435 pounds)
Let's now see what happens when this athlete lifts 425 pounds (1,934.98 newtons) with the high-bar back squat. With this technique, there is a more closed angle at the knee joint (now at 125 degrees compared to the previous 120 degrees with the low-bar technique). The angle at the hip joint will be at fifty-five degrees, which is more open when compared to the low-bar back squat hip angle of forty degrees. This is a normal change due to the more upright trunk position of this squat variation.[4]

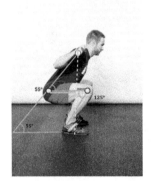

Torque = moment arm × force
   = 0.19 meters × 1,934.98 newtons
   = 367.6 NM or newton meters of force acting upon the knee joint at 125°

Torque = moment arm × force
   = 0.27 meters × 1,934.98 newtons
   = 522.4 NM or newton meters of force acting upon the hip joint and lumbar/pelvis complex at 55°

Front Squat Analysis (360 pounds)

Lastly, let's assume the same athlete now attempts to lift 378 pounds (1,681.43 newtons) with the front-squat technique. The angles during the freeze-frame at the parallel squat position will change again from the previous two techniques. The front squat uses a more closed angle of the knee joint (now at 130 degrees). It also employs a more vertical trunk in order to keep the bar balanced on the chest and centered over the middle of the foot. This opens up the hip joint and lower back to seventy-five degrees.

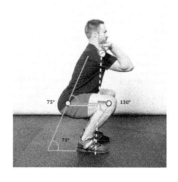

Torque = moment arm × force
 = 0.22 meters × 1,681.43 newtons
 = 369.9 NM or newton meters of force acting upon the knee joint at 130°

Torque = moment arm × force
 = 0.24 meters × 1,681.43 newtons
 = 403.5 NM or newton meters of force acting upon the hip joint and lumbar/pelvis complex at 75°

Comparative Analysis (Varying Weights across Techniques)
With this analysis, we can see some striking differences compared to the last investigation that evaluated each squat at the same weight.

- The low-bar back-squat technique placed dramatically more torque on the low back (lumbar/pelvis joint) and hip joint compared to the other techniques. In this parallel freeze-frame analysis, 717.7 newton meters of force were applied to the lower back and hip joint compared to the other techniques (522.4 newton meters in high-bar back squat and 403.5 newton meters in front squat). Comparatively, the low-bar squat placed 53 percent more torque on the hip and lower back than the high-bar squat and 78 percent more than the front squat.
- The low-bar back squat, however, placed the least amount of torque on the knee joint compared to the other techniques!

- The high-bar back squat placed relatively the same amount of torque on the knee joint as the front squat. Despite having a longer moment arm in the front squat and a more closed angle, the heavier weight of the back squat increased knee torque to the same level.

Final Thoughts

As you can see with this analysis, changing the weight on the bar can significantly change the amount of torque that is generated on the different joint complexes. The smallest change in variables (weight on the bar, technique used, etc.) can greatly change the forces placed on your body.

This allows us as coaches to make exercise recommendations for our athletes based on individual needs. For example, an athlete returning from a knee injury who can't yet tolerate a more forward knee position during a barbell squat would benefit from using a low-bar back squat compared to a high-bar variation. This is in part because more torque is placed on the knee joint during the high-bar back squat.

Also, an athlete dealing with back pain may benefit from using a front squat during training instead of the conventional back squat. This is because the front squat places less torque on the lower back compared to both back squat variations when more realistic weights are used. This recommendation is only practical if the injured athlete is able to perform the front squat with acceptable technique. An athlete with poor core control or restricted thoracic mobility may find it difficult to assume the form.

Exercise recommendations for healthy athletes' exercise

should not be based solely on the forces sustained at one joint. Research shows that healthy athletes can easily tolerate the forces for any of the three squat techniques.[7] You shouldn't worry about injuring the knee using high-bar or low-bar back squat. The ACL and other ligaments inside the knee joint should be completely safe. As long as good technique is used, joint stress values will never come close to exceeding harmful levels.[7]

Athletes should use a training program that employs multiple squat techniques to ensure a more balanced approach and to decrease risk of overuse injuries.

Notes

1. D. Diggin, C. O'Regan, N. Whelan, S. Daly, et al., "A Biomechanical Analysis of Front versus Back Squat: Injury Implications," *Portuguese Journal of Sport Sciences* 11, Suppl. 2 (2011): 643–46.
2. M. Rippetoe, *Starting Strength: Basic Barbell Training*, 3rd ed. (Wichita Falls, TX: The Aasgaard Company, 2011).
3. A. C. Fry, J. C. Smith, and B. K. Schilling, "Effect of Knee Position on Hip and Knee Torques during the Barbell Squat," *Journal of Strength and Conditioning Research* 17, no. 4 (2003): 629–33.
4. P. Wretenberg, Y. Feng, and U. P. Arborelius, "High- and Low-bar Squatting Techniques during Weight-training," *Medicine and Science in Sports and Exercise* 28, no. 2 (February 1996): 218–24.
5. P. O'Shea, "The Parallel Squat," *National Strength Conditioning Association Journal* 7 (1985): 4–6.
6. H. Hartmann, K. Wirth, and M. Klusemann, "Analysis of the Load on the Knee Joint and Vertebral Column with Changes in Squatting Depth and Weight Load," *Sports Medicine* 43, no. 10 (2013): 993–1008.
7. B. J. Schoenfeld, "Squatting Kinematics and Kinetics and Their Application to Exercise Performance," *Journal of Strength and Conditioning Research* 24, no. 12 (2010): 3497–506.

Acknowledgments

I heard a story once about a group of people who came across a turtle perched atop a fence post. A few among the group exclaimed, "Look at what this turtle has done! Only an expert climber could have made it this far!"

While this achievement was by all means extraordinary, there was *no way* the small turtle would have been capable of this feat all by itself. Someone *had* to help it reach his final destination.

This book is the accumulation of over three years of constant writing, editing, and rewriting. However, in the end, I know there is no way this book would have been possible without the help of so many people along the way.

First and foremost, I need to thank my wife, Christine. She has stood by my side and put up with my *constant* research and writing over these years. You are an angel, and I am thankful every day to have you by my side.

To my coauthor, Dr. Kevin Sonthana. This book would still be over five hundred pages and sound like a scientific research article if it wasn't for your input and vision. You have challenged me to become a better writer; for that, I am forever grateful.

To my mentor, Travis Neff. It has been a great privilege and honor to learn from such a hardworking and God-fearing man. The mantra "lead by example" is something you have modeled for me from the first day I started at Boost. Thank you so much for your contributions in writing and publishing this book.

To my current and past Olympic weightlifting coaches: Anna Martin, Dr. Tom LaFontaine, and Dr. Alex Koch. I cannot express enough thanks for the constant hours you have spent coaching and expanding my understanding of barbell training since 2005. Also, to the man who first taught me to pick up a barbell, coach Tom Sumner. Who would have thought that the skinny eighth-grader who walked into your weight room in 2000 would eventually grow up to write a book on squatting?

To my team members at Boost Physical Therapy & Sport Performance: especially Dr. Tyler Anderson, Ryan Ruble, David Rush, Ryan Johnson, Carissa Parker, and Emily Post. I feel truly blessed to work every day with others who share the same passions as I do!

To my best friends, Ryan Grout, Nate Varel, and Kevin Stock. Your input and support for this project have been priceless. One of the greatest gifts in this life is friendship, and I have truly received it.

To my parents, Dave and Jill. Thank you for the constant support you have provided my entire life. I can only aspire to be as good of a parent one day to my own children.

To my past professors at Truman State University and the University of Missouri. The education I received was second to none. Thank you.

A few books and authors have inspired me over the past years. These men have definitely changed my perspective on life: *Movement*, by Gray Cook; *Becoming a Supple Leopard*, by Dr. Kelly Starrett; *Starting Strength*, by Mark Rippetoe; *Start with*

Why, by Simon Sinek; *The Icon Effect*, by Darren Sugiyama; and *Crush It*, by Garry Vaynerchuk.

And finally, to all of those who try to live their life to the fullest each and every day. For those who live and teach the motto of "move *well* and *then* lift heavy." If enough of us realize and spread this message, we can truly change the world.

Aaron

CPSIA information can be obtained
at www.ICGtesting.com
Printed in the USA
LVHW030002020421
683199LV00004B/31